ID0984377

Fertility, Biology, and Behavior

*AN ANALYSIS OF
THE PROXIMATE DETERMINANTS*

This is a volume in

STUDIES IN POPULATION

A complete list of titles in this series appears at the end of this volume.

Fertility, Biology, and Behavior

AN ANALYSIS OF
THE PROXIMATE DETERMINANTS

John Bongaarts

Center for Policy Studies
Population Council
New York, New York

Robert G. Potter

Department of Sociology
Brown University
Providence, Rhode Island

ACADEMIC PRESS
A Subsidiary of Harcourt Brace Jovanovich, Publishers

New York London
Paris San Diego San Francisco São Paulo Sydney Tokyo Toronto

ACADEMIC PRESS, INC.
111 Fifth Avenue, New York, New York 10003

United Kingdom Edition published by
ACADEMIC PRESS, INC. (LONDON) LTD.
24/28 Oval Road, London NW1 7DX

Library of Congress Cataloging in Publication Data

Bongaarts, John, Date
    Fertility, Biology, and Behavior.

    Includes index.
    1. Fertility, Human. 2. Birth intervals. 3. Family
size. I. Potter, Robert G. II. Title. [DNLM:
1. Family planning . 2. Fertility. WP 565 B713f]
GN241.B66   1983   304.6'34   82-18435
ISBN 0-12-114380-5

PRINTED IN THE UNITED STATES OF AMERICA

83 84 85 86   9 8 7 6 5 4 3 2 1

Contents

1

Introduction and Overview

2

Natural Fertility and Its Proximate Determinants

3

Regulated Fertility and Its Proximate Determinants

4

An Aggregate Fertility Model

5

Applications of an Aggregate Fertility Model

6

A Macrosimulation Model and Applications to Fecundity and Natural Fertility

7

Family-Size Control

8

Birth Spacing

9

Sex Preselection

Preface

Human fertility has traditionally been investigated in two separate disciplines: biology and the social sciences. Reproductive physiologists have made extensive studies of the processes of ovulation, spermatogenesis and fertilization, and their regulation with contraceptive technology. Social scientists, on the other hand, have considered the number of children born to a woman to be largely an outcome of social norms, economic considerations, and cultural factors that shape the fertility control behavior of couples. A few early scholars—Raymond Pearl, Gilbert Beebe, and Regine Stix, for example—drew on both traditions, but their conceptual frames tended to be informal and eclectic. A more systematic approach was realized by the French demographer Louis Henry and the American sociologists Kingsley Davis and Judith Blake when they first identified the mechanisms through which socioeconomic processes and human behavior interact with the biological aspects of human reproduction. The biological and behavioral dimensions of human fertility are linked through a set of "proximate determinants" or "intermediate fertility variables." Examples of proximate determinants are the age at first marriage (controlling the onset of exposure to socially sanctioned childbearing), the use of contraception (to reduce or eliminate the probability of conceiving), and the breastfeeding duration and pattern (determining the length of the anovulation interval after a birth).

Most of the literature on the proximate determinants is scattered in a variety of journals and conference proceedings. Aside from a collection of Henry's early papers on the subject (*On the Measurement of Human Fertility,* Elsevier, 1972), only two books are available to summarize existing knowledge. In the first, *Mathematical Models of Conception and Birth* (University of Chicago Press, 1973), Sheps and Menken present a detailed and comprehensive discussion of reproductive models. Due to the technical nature of the material and extensive use of fairly advanced mathematical techniques, this excellent monograph is primarily of interest to biostatisticians and mathematical demographers. The second book, Leridon's *Human Fertility: The Basic Components* (University of Chicago Press, 1977), is much less technical and provides good reviews of the proximate determinants of natural fertility. The objective of this volume is to give an updated review of the proximate determinants and their effects on fertility, with special emphasis on important recent developments. The discussion of fertility models requires the introduction of some mathematical equations, but only simple equations are used here and their numbers are kept to an absolute minimum. Although the factors affecting natural fertility are reviewed, the principal focus will be on the proximate determinants of controlled fertility.

A substantial part of the material presented in the following chapters has been based on lecture notes used by the authors in teaching graduate courses in demography, sociology, and public health. However, the book is not only intended as a text for graduate students, but also as a reference for a broader audience of demographers, statisticians, social scientists, and biologists with an interest in the biological and behavioral control of human fertility.

Acknowledgments

Financial support for a substantial portion of the research presented in this volume was provided by Grants No. 5K04HD0037-02 and No. HD12100 from the National Institute of Child Health and Human Development and by Grant No. SES79-10326 from the National Science Foundation.

Permission to reprint parts of the following publications is gratefully acknowledged: "The supply of children: A critical essay," *Determinants of Fertility in Developing Countries*, National Academy of Sciences (forthcoming); "The proximate determinants of natural marital fertility," *Determinants of Fertility in Developing Countries*, National Academy of Sciences (forthcoming); "Estimating the impact of contraceptive prevalence on fertility: Aggregate and age specific versions of a model" in *The Role of Surveys in the Analysis of Family Planning Programs*, A. Hermalin and B. Entwisle, Eds., Ordina, Liege, 1982; "The fertility inhibiting effects of the intermediate fertility variables," *Analysis of Maternity Histories* (forthcoming); "A dynamic model of the reproductive process," *Population Studies*, 31, 1, 1977.

Quite indispensable were the programming services of Irene Gravel and Robert Sendek. A debt of gratitude is owed Carol Walker and Cynthia Freiman for their adept secretarial assistance.

1

Introduction and Overview

Studies of the causes of fertility trends and differentials often seek to measure directly the impact of socioeconomic factors on fertility. This approach has been used widely partly because measures of socioeconomic variables such as income, education, and place of residence are readily available and partly because policymakers in many countries are interested in identifying the factors that may be manipulated to influence fertility. Unfortunately, the results of these studies are far from conclusive. Not infrequently, relationships are found to differ not only in magnitude but even in direction in different settings and at different times (Cochrane 1979, Rodriguez and Cleland 1981).

To improve understanding of the causes of fertility variation it is necessary to analyze the mechanisms through which socioeconomic variables influence fertility. In response to this need demographers have turned to the study of the proximate determinants of fertility. The *proximate determinants* of fertility are the biological and behavioral factors through which social, economic, and environmental variables affect fertility. The principal characteristic of a proximate determinant is its direct influence on fertility. If a proximate determinant—such as contraceptive use—changes, then fertility necessarily changes also (assuming the other proximate determinants remain constant), though this is not necessarily the case for a socioeconomic determinant. Consequently, fertility differences among populations and trends in fertility over time can always be traced to variations in one or more of the proximate determinants. The following simple diagram summarizes the relationships among the determinants of fertility:

Social, economic, $\longrightarrow$ Proximate $\longrightarrow$ Fertility
environmental   determinants
factors

These relationships were first recognized in a now classical study by Davis and Blake (1956). Starting from the premise that reproduction involves the three necessary steps of intercourse, conception, and completion of gestation, Davis and Blake identified a set of 11 proximate determinants[1] which they called "intermediate fertility variables." A somewhat different approach to the analysis of the proximate determinants was taken by Henry (1953, 1957), who constructed the first detailed mathematical models of the reproductive process. Following this pioneering work, the investigation of the proximate determinants was pursued during the 1960s by a number of researchers, most notably Potter, Sheps, and Tietze. Much of their efforts focused on the construction of increasingly more realistic but sometimes highly complex models for the relationship between fertility and the proximate determinants. This development has continued into the 1980s and relatively simple yet quite realistic fertility models now exist. The construction of these models and their validation has been made possible by the greatly increased availability of empirical measures of the proximate variables in many populations. The resulting improvement in the understanding of the

---

[1] Davis and Blake (1956) proposed the following set of intermediate fertility variables:

I. Factors affecting exposure to intercourse ("intercourse variables")
   A. Those governing the formation and dissolution of unions in the reproductive period
      1. Age of entry into sexual unions
      2. Permanent celibacy: proportion of women never entering sexual unions
      3. Amount of reproductive period spent after or between unions
        a. When unions are broken by divorce, separation, or desertion
        b. When unions are broken by death of husband
   B. Those governing the exposure to intercourse within union
      4. Voluntary abstinence
      5. Involuntary abstinence (from impotence, illness, unavoidable but temporary separations)
      6. Coital frequency (excluding periods of abstinence).
II. Factors affecting exposure to conception ("conception variables")
      7. Fecundity or infecundity, as affected by involuntary causes
      8. Use or nonuse of contraception
        a. By mechanical and chemical means
        b. By other means
      9. Fecundity or infecundity, as affected by voluntary causes (sterilization, subincision, medical treatment, etc.)
III. Factors affecting gestation and successful parturition ("gestation variables")
      10. Fetal mortality from involuntary causes
      11. Fetal mortality from voluntary causes

fertility effects of the proximate variables has led to a more frequent inclusion of the proximate factors in studies of socioeconomic and environmental determinants of fertility (e.g., Bongaarts 1980, Cochrane 1979, Lesthaeghe, Shah, and Page 1981).

TERMINOLOGY

Before proceeding, it is useful to briefly discuss the basic terms, *fertility, fecundity,* and *fecundability.* Fertility refers to actual reproduction, whereas fecundity denotes the ability to reproduce. A woman who is bearing children is fertile; a woman is considered fecund if she is capable of bearing live offspring. The opposite terms are *infertility,* also called childlessness, and *infecundity,* which is synonymous with sterility. Sterility (or infecundity) implies the existence of infertility but the reverse is not necessarily the case. A fecund woman may choose to remain infertile by not marrying or by practicing highly effective contraception. Infertility then is either due to a voluntary decision not to have children or it is caused by (biological) infecundity.

The term fecundable refers to the ability to conceive. Fecund and fertile women are necessarily fecundable, although they may experience temporary periods of infecundability. However, some fecundable women are infecund, and consequently infertile, because they are physiologically unable to successfully complete a pregnancy. The term fecundability has taken on a specific meaning as the probability of conceiving per month (among cohabiting women who are not pregnant, sterile, or temporarily infecundable).

These definitions are given in the *Multilingual demographic dictionary* (United Nations, 1959) and are consistently used in the English demographic literature. It should be noted that in French and in other romance languages the terms fertility and fecundity are reversed; that is, fecondité is the equivalent of fertility and fertilité equals fecundity. To add further to the confusion, the words fertility and fecundity are used virtually synonymously in the biological and medical literature.

More specific meaning can be given to the terms fertility and fecundability by adding adjectives. For example, natural fertility is found in populations where no contraception or induced abortion is practiced; controlled or regulated fertility is observed in societies where fertility control practices are widespread. Similarly, natural fecundability is the monthly probability of conception in the absence of contraception, and residual or controlled fecundability refers to the conception risk in the presence of contraception.

THE PROXIMATE DETERMINANTS

Davis and Blake (1956) identified the first list of proximate determinants, but their set has not found wide acceptance in quantitative fertility studies because it is not easily incorporated into reproductive models. Extensions and variants of this set have been proposed by other researchers (e.g., Mosley 1978, Yaukey 1973). Model builders, however, have based their work largely on Henry's analysis of the reproductive process. This approach has produced a different, but closely overlapping, list of proximate determinants that has greatly simplified the task of constructing fertility models. It is this alternative set that will be presented here.

Figure 1.1 summarizes the various events that most immediately influence the duration of the reproductive period and the rate of childbearing during it. An examination of these events allows the identification of a complete set of proximate determinants. The potential reproductive years start at *menarche,* the first menstruation in a woman's life. Socially sanctioned childbearing, however, is in virtually all societies limited to women in relatively stable sexual unions. For convenience the term *marriage* will be used here to refer to all such unions. Marriage (or the first cohabitation) may in practice be taken as the starting point of the actual reproductive years, since it takes place, with few exceptions, after menarche. As a consequence, any changes in age at menarche can generally affect fertility only by influencing age at marriage. Once married, a woman may be considered at risk of childbearing until the onset of permanent sterility or menopause, unless a marital disruption intervenes. Childbearing can of course resume again after a marital disruption if the woman remarries.

While married and fecund, women reproduce at a rate inversely related to the average duration of the birth interval. Short birth intervals are associated with high fertility and vice versa. In the absence of intrauterine mortality, the

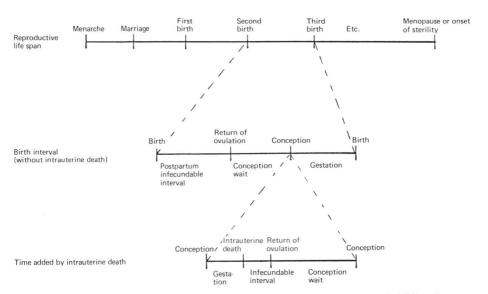

FIGURE 1.1.   Events determining the reproductive life span and the rate of childbearing.

length of a birth interval is determined by its three components (see Figure 1.1):

1. the postpartum infecundable interval. Immediately after a birth, a woman experiences an infecundable period during which the normal pattern of ovulation and menstruation is absent. The duration of this birth interval segment is primarily a function of breastfeeding behavior. (In a few societies, prolonged postpartum abstinence is practiced and the postpartum infecundable interval then exceeds the anovulatory interval to the extent that abstinence lasts beyond the resumption of ovulation.)

2. the waiting time to conception, also called the fecundable or ovulatory interval, from the first postpartum ovulation to conception. The length of this interval is inversely related to the natural fecundability (which, in turn, is largely determined by the frequency of intercourse) and to the use and effectiveness of contraception. Short conception delays are observed when natural fecundability is high and no contraception is practiced. The waiting time to conception lengthens with declining natural fecundability and with higher prevalence and effectiveness of contraception.

3. a full-term pregnancy. Because the duration of pregnancies ending in a live birth varies little, it is convenient to assume this birth interval segment to have a constant duration of 9 months.

In case a pregnancy ends prematurely in a spontaneous or induced intrauterine death, the birth interval is lengthened by the following additional components: a shortened pregnancy, a brief infecundable period, and a conception delay (see Figure 1.1).

In sum, this short review has identified the following seven proximate determinants: marriage (and marital disruption); onset of permanent sterility; postpartum infecundability; natural fecundability or frequency of intercourse; use and effectiveness of contraception; spontaneous intrauterine mortality; induced abortion.

The first two of these factors determine the duration of the reproductive period and the other five determine the rate of childbearing and the duration of birth intervals. The seven variables together constitute a complete set in the sense that socioeconomic and environmental factors can only affect fertility through one or more of these proximate variables.

FERTILITY AND THE PROXIMATE DETERMINANTS

As already noted, observed variations in fertility levels of populations are necessarily due to variations in one or more of the proximate determinants. How precisely the proximate determinants influence fertility will be discussed in detail in later chapters, but to introduce the subject, we will present here examples of fairly typical reproductive patterns in a few selected populations, including a modern developed, a traditional developing, and a histor-

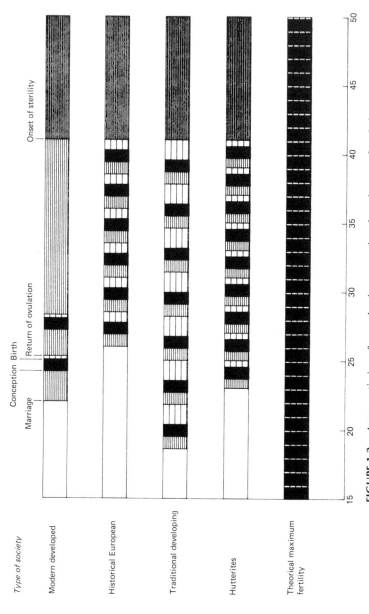

FIGURE 1.2. Average timing of reproductive events in selected types of societies.

ical European society. The results will then be compared with the fertility of the Hutterites and with the maximum level of reproduction that is theoretically possible. The average timing of reproductive events in these populations is summarized in Figure 1.2. To simplify this figure and the discussion of the findings, it is assumed that there is no marital disruption and the short period added to the average birth interval by spontaneous intrauterine mortality is included in the waiting time to conception.

A Modern Developed Society

In contemporary Western populations, women bear on average around two births during their reproductive years. A not unrepresentative timing of relevant events (summarized in Figure 1.2) would involve marriage in the early twenties and about 2 years between marriage and the first birth and 2 to 3 years between births. As the duration of postpartum infecundability is rather short, the spacing of the births is due to the use of contraception which prolongs the conception wait. The last child would be born in the middle to late twenties. To avoid having further births thereafter requires highly efficient contraceptive use or the practice of induced abortion until the onset of sterility, which on average occurs in the early forties.

A Historical European Population

In seventeenth- and eighteenth-century Europe, fertility was much higher than today, because little or no contraception or induced abortion was practiced. In a fairly typical case, women would average about six births between marriage in the mid-twenties and the end of the reproductive years. An average birth interval of around 2.5 years might consist of approximately equal segments for postpartum infecundability, conception delay, and gestation. Compared with the present, the age at marriage was later in the past and the duration of postpartum infecundability was longer because breastfeeding was more prevalent. Both factors would have caused a reduction in fertility. Fertility was nevertheless about three times higher then at present because these fertility-reducing effects are more than compensated by the absence of contraception, which is associated with an average waiting time to conception of well under a year.

A Traditional Developing Society

Over the past decades, the fertility of many of the least developed nations in Africa, Asia, and Latin America has remained relatively unchanged at about seven births per woman. In these societies, marriage usually takes place while the woman is in her teens and average birth intervals around 3 years are often observed. This average birth interval is longer than in most historical European populations because more prolonged and frequent breastfeeding causes longer periods of postpartum infecundability. Fertility is high despite these prolonged birth intervals because marriage takes place at an early age.

The Hutterites

The Hutterites are members of an Anabaptist sect descendent from Swiss settlers in the northern United States and in Canada. They live in small communities in which strict social and religious control exists over most aspects of daily life. Demographers have a strong interest in their society because the fertility rate of the Hutterites is higher than that of any other population with reliable records. In 1950, women who had reached the end of the childbearing years had born an average of about nine children (Eaton and Mayer 1953). Their high fertility was made possible by spacing births about 2 years apart throughout their reproductive years, beginning with marriage in their early twenties. The average birth interval of the Hutterites is substantially shorter than in traditional-developing countries because breastfeeding is less prolonged so that their period of postpartum infecundability is only about 6 months.

Theoretical Maximum Fertility

Although the Hutterites have the highest observed fertility rate, it could theoretically be much higher. Reproduction can start in the mid-teens and can continue until near age 50. In addition, birth intervals lasting 1 year or even less are biologically possible because a full-term gestation takes only 9 months. Theoretically then, in the absence of all biological and behavioral constraints on reproduction, a woman could have 35 births (not counting multiple births) between ages 15 and 50, if birth intervals were to average one year. Hutterite fertility is far short of this biological maximum for several reasons, including delayed marriage, the practice of breastfeeding, a moderate frequency of intercourse, a substantial risk of intrauterine mortality, and the onset of sterility of either the male or female in the early forties.

An alternative way to summarize the reproductive patterns of these five populations is presented in Table 1.1., which gives the average proportions of the reproductive years spent in various reproductive states. Five reproductive states are distinguished:

Table 1.1
APPROXIMATE PERCENTAGE OF THE POTENTIAL REPRODUCTIVE YEARS (15–50) SPENT IN DIFFERENT REPRODUCTIVE STATES IN SELECTED TYPES OF SOCIETIES

		Reproductive states			
Society	Single	Postpartum infecundable	Fecundable	Pregnant	Sterile
1. Developed	20	1	49	4	26
2. Historical European	31	15	15	13	26
3. Contemporary developing	10	30	19	15	26
4. Hutterites	23	13	19	19	26
5. Theoretical maximum fertility	0	16	9	75	0

1. Single
2. Postpartum infecundable
3. Fecundable (including time added by spontaneous intrauterine mortality)
4. Pregnant before a live birth
5. Permanently sterile

The estimates in Table 1.1 should be considered illustrative, especially as no allowance is made for marital disruption. Except in the hypothetical case with biological maximum fertility, about a quarter of the potential reproductive years between ages 15 and 50 is, on average, spent in the sterile state. This is caused by the fact that the average age at onset of sterility is in the early forties (see Chapter 2). As expected, the time in the pregnant state rises proportionately with the level of fertility (total fertility rates are assumed to be 2, 6, 7, 9, and 35 respectively in the five populations in Table 1.1). No clear pattern emerges in the estimates of the time in the three remaining reproductive states. It is noteworthy that women in contemporary developed societies are fecundable for nearly half of their reproductive years. This is the consequence of the widespread use of contraception that reduces fecundability to a fraction of its natural level.

VARIATIONS IN INDIVIDUAL FERTILITY

The description of fertility patterns in the preceeding section dealt strictly with the population averages of the timing of reproductive events. In reality, few women bear children at the regular average rate outlined in Figure 1.2. Not only does the timing of reproductive events differ substantially among women, but there is also wide variation in the number of births women have. This is clear from Figure 1.3, which plots the distribution of the number of

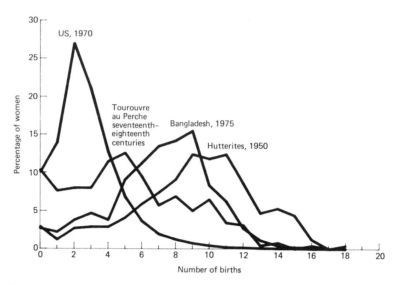

FIGURE 1.3. Distribution of percentage of ever-married women at the end of the reproductive years, by number of children ever born, in selected populations.

past births among ever-married women at the end of the reproductive years in selected populations. In each of these four cases, the number of children ever born ranges from 0 to well over 10, although there are admittedly few of these high-parity women in the United States as of 1970. The other three examples are from populations with natural fertility. Their parity distributions have a large standard deviation and fewer than one in six women had the modal number of births.

As in the aggregate case, variations in the fertility of individual women are caused by variations in the proximate determinants. In the United States and other modern societies one can expect to find differences in the number of children born because the desired family size varies among women and contraception is available to help achieve these objectives. In addition, some women will have fewer or more than the desired number of births for non-voluntary reasons, such as the premature onset of sterility or contraceptive failure. (This topic will be explored in detail in Chapter 7.)

In natural fertility populations, contraception and induced abortion are virtually absent, and the remaining proximate variables must, therefore, be responsible for the large variances of the parity distributions shown in Figure 1.3. In fact, both the duration of the reproductive years and the length of birth intervals vary widely among women. As an example, the distributions of the age at first marriage and the age at the onset of permanent sterility in Tourouvre au Perche, in the seventeenth and eighteenth century, (Charbonneau 1970) are plotted in the upper panel of Figure 1.4. The age at first marriage ranged from below 20 to over 40, and the age of onset of sterility had an equally large range. As a consequence, the number of years actually available for childbearing ranged from 0 for the women (couples) who were sterile at marriage to over 30 for those who married early and remained fecund until their late forties. The former will by necessity have no offspring whereas the latter have a good chance of bearing more than 10 children.

The duration of the birth interval is also highly variable. The distribution of the interval between first and second births in Tourouvre au Perche, plotted in the lower panel of Figure 1.4, shows that the length of birth intervals ranged from less than 1 year to over 4 years. Systematic differences in breastfeeding behavior, frequency of intercourse, and risk of spontaneous intrauterine mortality are major causes of this finding, but an important random element is also present (see Chapter 6 for details). For example, the

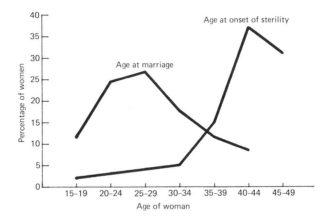

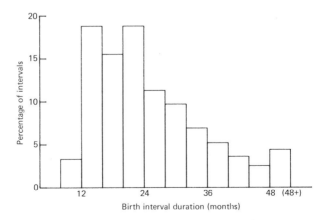

FIGURE 1.4. Distribution of age at first marriage and age at onset of permanent sterility, and the distribution of the interval between first and second births for Tourouvre au Perche, seventeenth and eighteenth centuries.

conception delay would still be highly variable even if couples all had the same frequency of intercourse because conception depends on unpredictable events such as the exact timing of ovulation and the successful implantation of the fertilized ovum. Similarly, some women may experience no spontaneous abortions, whereas others have several despite a biologically equal risk of a spontaneous intrauterine death. As will be shown in Chapter 8, the intrinsically stochastic nature of the reproductive process prevents the exact prediction or control of the timing of births.

AGE-SPECIFIC FERTILITY

Fertility varies with the woman's age in all human societies for which measurements exist. The rate of childbearing is lowest in the youngest and oldest age groups, and fertility reaches a maximum in the central-childbearing years. The causes of this variation are the age patterns in the proximate determinants. For example, the marriage pattern is of major importance in explaining the shape of the age-specific fertility curve because the proportion married varies substantially with age. This proportion is lowest in the 15- to 19-year-old age group, and it is, therefore, one of the principal reasons for the relatively low fertility rate of this age group. The proportions married usually decline in the older age groups as the effects of marital disruption cumulate, thus contributing to the reduction of fertility rates toward the end of the childbearing years.

Even though the marriage pattern has a major impact on the age pattern of fertility, the other proximate determinants also have an effect. This is evident from the changes with age in the fertility of married women. Two examples of age-specific marital fertility rates—one from the United States and the other from the Hutterites—are plotted in Figure 1.5. In both cases, marital fertility declines after age 20. The differences between the United States and the Hutterite levels of marital fertility are almost entirely due to differences in the practice of contraception and induced abortion. (This conclusion is based on findings presented in Chapters 2 and 4 which show that the incidence of sterility and the risk of spontaneous intrauterine mortality vary little among populations and that the slightly longer postpartum infecundability of the Hutterite women is largely compensated by a shorter natural waiting time before conception.)

Hutterite women use virtually no contraception or induced abortion, and the age pattern in their marital fertility rates must consequently be caused by the four remaining proximate determinants: sterility, postpartum infecundability, natural fecundability, and spontaneous intrauterine mortality. Unfortunately, direct age-specific measures of these factors are not available. However, a standard age-specific sterility pattern proposed by Henry (1965) may be applied as a good approximation because populations differ little in

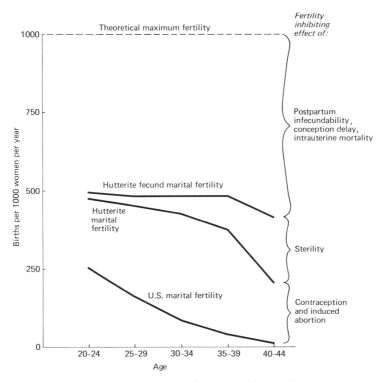

FIGURE 1.5.   Age-specific marital fertility rates of the United States (1967) and Hutterites (marriages 1921–1930), and estimated age-specific marital fertility rates of fecund Hutterite women.

their prevalence of natural sterility (see Chapter 2). By dividing the age-specific marital fertility rates by the nonsterile proportion in each age group, we obtain estimates of the age-specific marital fertility rates of the fecund Hutterites. The results are also plotted in Figure 1.5. There is only a modest decline with age in the fertility rate of married fecund women. This finding indicates that the sterility pattern is an important determinant of the marital fertility schedule. It also suggests that any age-related increase in the risk of intrauterine mortality, decline in frequency of intercourse, and rise in postpartum infecundability have together only a modest impact on the age pattern of fertility. This conclusion does not imply that these three proximate variables are not important determinants of the overall level of fertility. In fact, they are the reason that the fecund marital fertility rate averages only about 500 rather than the theoretical maximum of a 1000 births per 1000 women per year.

Only fecund women bear offspring. The average birth interval is therefore inversely related to the age-specific fecund marital fertility rate in populations with natural fertility. For example, the average birth interval of the

Hutterites was earlier estimated to be 2 years; this duration is consistent with the average fecund marital fertility rate of about 500 births per 1000 women per year (or .5 births per women per year) found in Figure 1.5.

THE DETERMINANTS OF THE PROXIMATE VARIABLES

Socioeconomic factors and health and nutrition are the determinants of the proximate variables. As will be seen, health and nutrition are, in general, relatively unimportant determinants of fertility. Socioeconomic factors must therefore be the principal causes of fertility trends and differentials. A discussion of this topic is outside the scope of this book, but it should be noted that there is no general agreement on how socioeconomic and cultural factors operate to affect the proximate determinants and fertility. Reviews are available elsewhere (e.g., Andorka 1978, Cassen 1976, Freedman 1975, Hawthorn 1970, International Research Awards Program 1981, Miro and Potter 1980, National Academy of Sciences 1982, United Nations 1973). Although social scientists and demographers have studied the socioeconomic determinants of fertility for some time, relatively little attention has been given to the potential effects of nutrition and health. A short overview of this subject follows.

Nutrition

Frisch (1975, 1978) has suggested that malnutrition inhibits reproductive performance by delaying menarche and reducing the age at menopause, and by causing increases in the incidence of anovulatory cycles, the risk of spontaneous intrauterine mortality, and the duration of postpartum amenorrhea. This hypothesis has stimulated a growing number of investigations designed to establish its validity. The results of these studies are summarized in three reviews of the evidence (Bongaarts 1980, Gray 1982, Menken, Trussell, and Watkins 1981). The current consensus is that moderate chronic malnutrition such as prevails in many poor developing countries has only a very minor influence on fertility. On the other hand, the acute starvation found in famines causes a substantial reduction in fertility. The weak effect of chronic malnutrition apparently operates primarily through two of the proximate variables: the age at marriage as affected by the timing of menarche, and the duration of postpartum infecundability.

Several types of direct and indirect evidence indicate that malnutrition is associated with a higher age of menarche (Bongaarts 1980):

1. In contemporary developed countries, the mean age at menarche is near 13 years, whereas it is generally higher in the developing countries (e.g.,

13–14 in India and 15.7 in Bangladesh). Estimates for nineteenth-century European populations are also high—around 16 years

2. In one U.S. study, well-nourished girls reached menarche 2 years earlier than undernourished girls (Frisch 1972)

3. Nutritional status as measured by anthropometric indicators, such as body weight, are positively correlated with the probability of reaching menarche by a given age

4. In Western societies with relatively reliable historical data on age at menarche, a decline in age at menarche of about 3 years has taken place since the end of the last century. This decline is associated with an increase in body size and an improved diet

5. Socioeconomic status and age at menarche are negatively related in a number of countries. Differences ranging from a few months to about 2 years have been found between urban and rural populations and between high- and low-income groups.

Although there can be little doubt that malnutrition is associated with later age of menarche, the demographic impact of this effect can be shown to be quite small. Age at menarche signals the beginning of potential childbearing, but actual reproduction starts at marriage. The mean age at marriage is almost always higher than the mean age at menarche. The difference ranges from about 2 years in some traditional societies to more than 10 years in a number of contemporary populations. In populations where the mean age at marriage is near 20 or higher, one can hardly expect a fertility effect from nutritional variations in age at menarche, whereas the effect on the total fertility rate is only of the order of 5% following a large change in nutrition, even if marriage takes place shortly after menarche and if ages of the two events are correlated (Bongaarts 1980).

In discussing the relationship between nutrition and lactational infecundability, it is important to make a distinction between changes in maternal and infant nutrition. As will be seen in Chapter 2, the provision of dietary supplements to a nursing infant shortens the interval of lactational anovulation because the intensity of breastfeeding declines. The question of interest here is whether the duration of lactational infecundability is influenced by the maternal nutritional status if breastfeeding behavior remains unchanged. Studies in Bangladesh and Guatemala provide tentative estimates of the importance of moderate chronic malnutrition. Women were divided into groups of high, medium, and low nutritional status on the basis of anthropometric measures. The difference in the duration of lactational infecundability between the groups of high and low nutritional status were 1.1 and 1.0 months in the two studies in Bangladesh (Huffman, Chowdhury, Chakborty, & Mosley, 1978, Chowdhury 1978) and 1.6 months in Guatemala (Bongaarts and Delgado 1979). Only the latter difference was statistically significant. It should be noted that these analyses did not control for the duration of lactation. It is unlikely, however, that this substantially affects the results because women in these countries usually breastfeed their infants until the next pregnancy occurs, and, for nearly all women, ovulation resumes during lactation. A direct comparison of the relative importance of breastfeeding duration and nutritional intake as determinants of amenorrhea is available for a Guatemalan population (Delgado, Lechtig, Brineman, Martorell, Yarbrough, & Klein 1978). The results presented in Table 1.2 clearly indicate that the duration of lactation is the primary determinant. There is a fairly consistent, but not statistically significant, difference of the order of 1 month between the amenorrhea periods of women with high and low caloric intake. A nutritionally induced variation of the order of 1 month would result in a difference of only a few percentage points between the total fertility rates of well- and poorly nourished groups of women because this change in duration of lactational infecundability represents only a small fraction of the typically average birth interval of 2.5 to 3 years in this population.

The small differences in the durations of amenorrhea of nutritional status groups are not necessarily caused by a direct physiological effect of malnutrition on the mother. It is possible that unmeasured differences in the pattern of breastfeeding between the poorly and well-nourished women in these populations are responsible. For example, if malnourished mothers have less food available for supplementing infant diets, or are later in introducing supplementation, then their infants would require more intense breastfeeding, thus prolonging amenorrhea.

In contrast to the apparently small effects of chronic moderate malnutrition, acute starvation causes drastic reductions in fertility. Famines are in-

Table 1.2

MEAN DURATION OF POSTPARTUM AMENORRHEA (MONTHS) IN GROUPS DIFFERING IN CALORIC INTAKE AND IN DURATION OF LACTATION (NUMBER IN PARENTHESES)[a]

Daily caloric intake [b]	Duration of lactation (months)			
	7 - 12	13 - 18	19 - 24	25 or more
Low	6.54(13)	12.03(35)	16.44(45)	19.93(14)
Middle	6.31(13)	11.64(33)	15.47(57)	18.90(10)
High	5.47(14)	11.13(30)	14.60(47)	19.64(11)
High-low difference	1.07	0.90	1.84	0.29

[a] From Delgado, Lechtig, Brineman, Martorell, Yarbrough and Klein (1978).

[b] Low caloric intake = <1309 calories a day; middle = 1309 - 1630 calories; high = >1630 calories.

variably followed by large but temporary reductions in fertility 9 months later. The exact causes of this decline remain to be determined, but several factors are involved. It is evident that fecundity is impaired during a famine because a substantial proportion of women become amenorrheic. It is not clear, however, whether this amenorrhea is entirely due to malnutrition or is in part caused by the fear of death and the anxiety that accompanies the crisis. Psychological stress alone can induce amenorrhea. Other factors that may contribute to the decline in fertility during a famine are the separation of spouses in the search for food or work, a decline in libido, and voluntary birth control through contraception, induced abortion, or abstinence. A lack of sufficiently detailed data makes it impossible to estimate accurately the contributions from each of these factors. They would in any case vary in their impact in different famines.

Health

In a review of the available evidence, Gray (1982) concluded that general poor health is unlikely to have a substantial impact on fecundity because morbidity severe enough to inhibit reproduction afflicts only a minority of the disadvantaged women. An important exception to this generalization is the relatively high prevalence of pathological sterility in a few populations, primarily in parts of tropical Africa. The apparent cause of this sterility is pelvic inflammatory disease which in most cases is the consequence of sexually transmitted infections such as gonorrhea (Gray 1982).

In addition to the minor direct effect of poor health on reproductive capacity, there are two indirect effects of improved health on fertility. The first is the result of the lengthening of breastfeeding and postpartum infecundability as infant mortality declines. An infant death interrupts breastfeeding, but with fewer such deaths these interruptions will occur less frequently. The second indirect effect of changing health operates through a decline in the risk of widowhood. As adult mortality declines, so does the incidence of widowhood. The extent of the resulting increase in the proportions married in a population depends on the remarriage frequency. If most widows remarry quickly then a change in adult mortality would have little effect on overall fertility, but in the absence of remarriage, the impact can be substantial. It should be noted that the two indirect effects of improved health and mortality tend to compensate one another. That is, improved infant mortality and the consequent lengthening of the birth interval causes a reduction in the total fertility rate, whereas a decline in widowhood would raise it. In fact, in one simulation of fertility patterns characteristic of the population of India by Ridley, Sheps, and Menken (1967), it was found that the combined impact of these two indirect effects was very small.

THE ORGANIZATION OF THIS BOOK

Chapters 2 and 3 are largely descriptive in nature. A summary of present knowledge of the proximate determinants of natural marital fertility—postpartum infecundability, natural fecundability, spontaneous intrauterine mortality, and permanent sterility—is provided first, followed by a overview of levels, trends, and differentials of the proximate determinants of controlled fertility—marriage, contraception, and induced abortion—in selected populations. Chapters 4 and 5 present a detailed analysis of a simple, aggregate reproductive model that quantifies the relationships between fertility and its proximate determinants. After describing and testing the model, it is used in a series of applications to gain insights into the operation of the proximate determinants and to solve specific problems.

In contrast to this first part of the monograph, which focuses on aggregate and average patterns of reproduction, the second part emphasizes individual variation in fertility patterns including the important role played by chance factors in this variation. A simulation model well adapted to trace variation among couples is described in an initial section of Chapter 6. The model is then employed to evaluate the scatter of family sizes occurring under conditions of natural fertility and fecundity. Chapter 7 considers to what extent delayed marriage, intentional postponement of childbearing in marriage, and the deliberate spacing of desired births elevate the risk of not attaining desired family size at all. It also assesses the effectiveness of contraception and the amounts of induced abortion and sterilization necessary to achieve prefigured levels of control over excess fertility. Chapter 8 evaluates to what extent regulation of birth timing may be improved by raising natural fecundability together with appropriate decisions about when to interrupt contraception. Chapter 9 deals with controlling the sex composition of children, principally through the use of amniocentesis and selective abortion.

The last four chapters are of a more technical character than the first five and include detailed descriptions of particular applications of reproductive models. The general reader might be well advised in his or her first reading to consult the introductions and summaries of Chapters 6–9 before deciding which working parts of these chapters to delve into.

REFERENCES

Andorka, R. (1978), *Determinants of Fertility in Advanced Societies,* The Free Press, New York.

Bongaarts, J. (1980), "Does Malnutrition Affect Fecundity? A Summary of Evidence," *Science,* 208, 565–569.

Bongaarts, J. and H. Delgado (1979), "Effects of Nutritional Status on Fertility in Rural Guatemala," in *Patterns and Determinants of Natural Fertility,"* H. Leridon and J. Menken, Eds., Ordina, Liege.

Cassen, R. H. (1976), "Population and Development: A Survey," *World Development, 4*,
    10–11, 785–830.
Charbonneau, H. (1970), "Tourouvre-au-Perche aux XVII et SVIII Siecles," INED, Travaux et
    Documents, Cahier No. 55, Presses Universitaires de France, Paris.
Chowdhury, A. K. N. (1978). "Effect of Maternal Nutrition on Fertility in Rural Bangladesh,"
    in *Nutrition and Human Reproduction,* W. M. Mosley, Ed., Plenum Press, New York.
Cochrane, S. H. (1979), "Fertility and Education. What Do we Really Know?" World Bank
    Staff Occasional Papers, No. 26, The Johns Hopkins University Press, Baltimore.
Davis, K. and J. Blake (1956), "Social Structure and Fertility: An Analytic Framework,"
    Economic Development and Cultural Change, 4, 4, 211–235.
Delgado, H., A. Lechtig, E. Brineman, R. Martorell, C. Yarbrough, and R. E. Klein, (1978),
    "Nutrition and Birth Interval Components: The Guatemalan Experience," in *Nutrition
    and Human Reproduction,* W. M. Mosley, Ed., Plenum Press, New York.
Eaton, J. W. and A. J. Mayer (1953), "The Social Biology or Very High Fertility Among the
    Hutterites: The Demography of a Unique Population," *Human Biology, 25,* 3, 206–264.
Freedman, R. (1975), *The Sociology of Human Fertility,* Irvington Publishers, New York.
Frisch, R. E. (1972), "Weight at Menarche: Similarity for Well-Nourished and Undernourished
    Girls at Different Ages and Evidence of Historical Constancy, *Pediatrics, 50,* 445–450.
Frisch, R. E. (1975), "Demographic Implications of the Biological Determinants of Female
    Fecundity," *Social Biology, 22,* 1, 17–22.
Frisch, R. E. (1978), "Population, Food Intake and Fertility," *Science, 199* (6 January), 22–30.
Gray, R. (1982), "Factors Affecting Natural Fertility Components: Health and Nutrition," in
    Determinants of Fertility in Developing Countries, National Academy of Sciences (in
    press).
Hawthorn, G. (1970), *The Sociology of Fertility,* Collier-MacMillan, London.
Henry, L. (1953), "Fondements Theoriques des Mesures de la Fecondite Naturelle," *Review de
    L'Institut International de Statistique, 21,* 3, 135–252. Translated in *On the Measurement
    of Human Fertility,* Elsevier, Amsterdam (1972).
Henry, L. (1957), "Fecondite et Famille, Models Mathematiques," *Population, 12,* 3, 413–444.
    Translated in *On the Measurement of Human Fertility,* Elsevier, Amsterdam (1972).
Henry, L. (1961), "Some Data on Natural Fertility," *Eugenics Quarterly, 8,* 2, 81–91.
Henry, L. (1965), "French Statistical Research in Natural Fertility," in *Pulic Health and
    Population Change,* M. C. Sheps and J. C. Ridley, Eds., University of Pittsburgh Press,
    Pittsburgh.
Henry, L. (1972), *On the Measurement of Human Fertility,* M. C. Sheps and E. Lapierre-
    Adamyck, Eds., Elsevier, New York.
Hodgson, M. and J. Gibbs (1980), "Children Ever Born," Comparative Studies, Cross National
    Summaries, No. 12. World Fertility Survey, London.
Huffman, S. L., A. M. U. Chowdhury, I. Chakborty, and W. H. Mosley (1978), "Nutrition and
    Postpartum Amenorrhea in Rural Bangladesh," *Population Studies, 32,* 2, 251–260.
International Research Awards Program (1981), "Research on the Determinants of Fertility: A
    Note on Priorities," *Population and Development Review, 7,* 2 311–323.
Leridon, H. (1977), *Human Fertility: The Basis Components.* The University of Chicago Press,
    Chicago.
Lesthaeghe, R. J., I. H. Shah and H. J. Page (1981), "Compensating Changes in Intermediate
    Fertility Variables and the Onset of Natural Fertility Transition," in Proceedings of the
    IUSSP General Conference, Manila, Ordina, Liege.
Menken, J., J. Trussell and S. Watkins (1981), "The Nutrition-Fertility Link: An Evaluation of
    the Evidence," *Journal of Interdisciplinary History, 9,* 425–441.
Miro, L. A. and J. E. Potter (1980), *Population Policy: Research Priorities in the Developing
    World,* Francis Pinter, London.
Mosley, W. M. (1978), "Issues, Definitions and an Analytic Framework," in *Nutrition and
    Human Reproduction,* W. M. Mosley, Ed., Plenum Press, New York.

National Academy of Sciences (1982), *The Determinants of Fertility in Developing Countries: A Summary of Knowledge*, Report of the Panel on Fertility Determinants, (forthcoming).

Ridley, J., M. Sheps, J. Linger and J. Menken (1967), "The Effects of Changing Mortality on Natality," *Milbank Memorial Fund Quarterly*, 45, 77–97.

Rodriguez, G. and J. Cleland (1981), "Socioeconomic Determinants of Marital Fertility in Twenty Countries: A Multivariate Analysis," *World Fertility Survey Conference* 1980, Record of Proceedings, International Statistical Institute, Voorburg, Netherlands.

Sheps, M. C. and J. A. Menken (1973), *Mathematical Models of Conception and Birth*, University of Chicago Press, Chicago.

United Nations (1959), Multilingual Demographic Dictionary, Population Studies, No. 29, United Nations, New York.

United Nations (1973), "The Determinants and Consequences of Population Trends," Department of Economic and Social Affairs, Population Studies, No. 50, United Nations, New York.

U.S. Bureau of the Census (1973), "Women by Number of Children Ever Born," Census of Population 1970, Subject Reports, No. PC(2)-3A, U.S. Government Printing Office, Washington, D.C.

Yaukey, D. (1973), *Marriage Reduction and Fertility*, Lexington, Massachusetts.

2

Natural Fertility and Its Proximate Determinants

NATURAL FERTILITY

Natural fertility is defined by Henry (1961) as fertility in the absence of deliberate birth control that is "bound to the number of children already born and is modified when the number exceeds the maximum which the couple does not wish to exceed [p. 81]." In practice, fertility may be considered natural if no contraception or induced abortion is used (Henry 1979). Most populations are at or near their natural level of fertility before the onset of the fertility transition. For example, societies with high and stable fertility in the contemporary developing world are governed by fertility regimens close to natural, especially in the rural and uneducated classes. Henry admits that the adjective "natural" is not an ideal one, but he prefers the term natural fertility over physiological or biological fertility because there are a number of nonbiological factors that have an important influence on natural fertility. Practices such as prolonged breastfeeding (which tends to inhibit ovulation) or postpartum abstinence lower fertility to well below its biological maximum, yet they are considered natural if they are not deliberately modified as the number of children already born rises. Natural fertility is further reduced in all human societies by delayed marriage and marital disruption.

A society's level of natural fertility is determined by its marriage pattern and by its level of natural marital fertility. Both these factors vary widely among populations, but empirical research in different societies with natural fertility has demonstrated that age pattern of marital fertility is relatively invariant (Coale and Trussel 1974, Henry 1961, Knodel 1977, 1981). Regardless of the overall level, age-specific natural marital rates show a very similar decline with age. For example, there is a substantial difference between the marital fertility of the Hutterites and of women in Nepal, but the age patterns are nearly the same (see Figure 2.1). On the basis of this finding, Coale and Trussell (1974, p. 188) have proposed a standard schedule of natural marital fertility that yields the following relative age pattern:

Age	Relative marital fertility level
20–24	100
25–29	94
30–34	86
35–39	70
40–44	36
45–49	5

Figure 2.1 shows that the convex shape of the natural fertility pattern is very different from the concave shape that characterizes societies such as the United States in which deliberate parity-dependent birth control is exerted

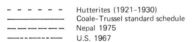

- - - - - - Hutterites (1921–1930)
—————— Coale-Trussel standard schedule
— — — — — Nepal 1975
—··—··—··— U.S. 1967

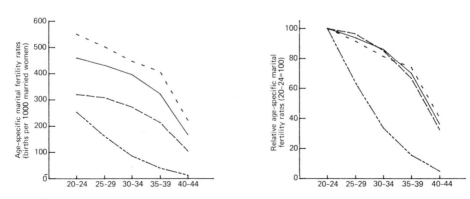

FIGURE 2.1. Absolute and relative age-specific marital fertility rates of selected populations.

through the use of contraception and/or induced abortion. This striking difference between the age patterns of natural and controlled marital fertility has allowed the identification of natural fertility populations solely on the basis of the shape of age-specific marital fertility rates (Coale and Trussell 1974, Knodel 1977).

The attention given in the literature to the constancy of the natural age pattern of marital fertility may have given the impression to some observers that overall levels of natural fertility are also relatively invariant. In fact, there is a great deal of variation in natural fertility. In a review of levels of natural fertility in 23 populations, Leridon (1977) found that the total fertility rate ranged from 3.7 in the french village of Thezels Saint-Sernin (marriages 1700–1791) to 9.5 among the Hutterites (marriages 1921–1930). Even this highest reliably observed fertility of the Hutterites is still restrained by delayed marriage (the median age at first marriage of females is 22) and by breastfeeding (the average duration of lactational amenorrhea is about 6 months). It has been estimated that natural fertility can reach around 15 births per woman if the fertility inhibiting effects of delayed marriage, marital disruption, and breastfeeding are also removed (Bongaarts 1978).

As was indicated in Chapter 1, the variation in levels of natural fertility can be explained by the effects of a set of fertility-inhibiting proximate determinants of fertility that exist in all societies but vary in their impact. Five proximate determinants of natural fertility were identified: the proportion of women married, the duration of postpartum infecundability, (natural) fecundability, the risk of intrauterine mortality, and the onset of permanent sterility. The last four variables are the proximate determinants of natural marital fertility which will be discussed in the next section. Directly related factors such as the breast-feeding effect on postpartum infecundability and the influence of frequency of intercourse on (natural) fecundability will also be reviewed here. Although it is an important proximate determinant of natural fertlity, the marriage pattern will not be discussed until Chapter 3.

THE PROXIMATE DETERMINANTS OF NATURAL MARITAL FERTILITY

Postpartum Infecundability

The first clear indication that periods of postpartum infecundability are demographically important were found in birth histories of women in historical societies with natural fertility. In these populations, the interval between marriage and first birth was, on average, substantially shorter than the interval between first and second births (Gautier and Henry 1958, Henripin, 1954). A plausible explanation for this difference in duration is the existence of an infecundable interval following a birth (but not marriage) because both intervals contain gestation and ovulatory segments of approximately the same duration, and conceptions are subject to similar risks of intrauterine mortality (Henry 1964). Consistent with this finding is the effect of an infant death on the birth interval. When an infant survives, the birth interval is on average longer than when an infant dies. Moreover, the earlier the death takes place, the shorter the birth interval is (Cantrelle and Leridon 1971, Henripin 1954, Knodel 1968, Potter, Wyon, New, and Gordon 1965). Henry (1964) concluded that the death of an infant either ends the anovulatory interval because breastfeeding is terminated, or causes the resumption of sexual relations in societies with a postpartum taboo against intercourse.

Direct measurements of the postpartum anovulatory or amenorrhea interval are now available in a number of populations (see the next section on "Breastfeeding and Postpartum Amenorrhea" for a discussion). Very prolonged amenorrhea periods have been observed, ranging up to 2 years in some societies. These long intervals of infecundability exert a powerful fertility-inhibiting effect because a large proportion (up to half) of the women's reproductive years are spent in the amenorrheic state. Most studies on the subject do not estimate the anovulatory interval directly, but instead measure the interval from birth to the first postpartum menses, a fairly well-defined event that is easier to measure. Some earlier investigators added one or two anovulatory cycles to the observed duration of postpartum amenorrhea to obtain an estimate of the total duration of postpartum anovulation, but this is now considered unnecessary. In the large majority of women, the first ovulation takes place within a few weeks before or after the first postpartum menses (Pascal 1969, Perez, Vela, Potter, and Masnick 1971). The mean duration of amenorrhea is therefore a good indicator of the mean duration of anovulation. The fact that ovulation often takes place before the resumption of the menses implies that women who engage in intercourse without contraception are at risk of conceiving while still amenorrheic. Data from several populations indicate that up to about 7% of women conceive without having menstruated (Van Ginneken 1978).

In most societies the duration of postpartum infecundability equals the duration of amenorrhea (or anovulation) because little or no postpartum abstinence is practiced. However, in a few populations, postpartum abstinence is practiced widely and for prolonged periods, resulting in abstinence intervals that exceed the amenorrhea intervals of many women. For example in parts of western Africa, strict taboos against intercourse during breastfeeding exist and average abstinence intervals up to 3 years have been observed (Caldwell and Caldwell 1977, Page and Lesthaeghe 1981).

Breastfeeding and Postpartum Amenorrhea

The temporary absence of menstruation after a birth is often called lactational amenorrhea because it is now well established that breastfeeding is the principal determinant of amenorrhea. Without breastfeeding the average amenorrhea interval is short—usually 1.5–2 months (Leridon 1977). With increasing duration of breastfeeding, the duration of amenorrhea rises, although not at the same rate. That is, an additional month of breastfeeding increases amenorrhea, on average, by less than one month. This is demonstrated in the upper panel of Table 2.1 which presents estimates of the average breastfeeding and amenorrhea intervals in a number of populations. A similar relationship between breastfeeding and amenorrhea is observed when one compares groups of women with different durations of breastfeeding in the same population. A typical example from Taiwan is given in the lower panel of Table 2.1. In this population both the breastfeeding and amenorrhea intervals vary widely among women, but there is a clear, positive relationship between these intervals. Similar strong positive correlations between the mean durations of breastfeeding and amenorrhea of subgroups have been reported in Senegal (Cantrelle and Leridon, 1971), in Guatemala (Delgado, Lechtig, Brineman, Martorell, Yarbrough, and Klein 1978), in the Philippines (Osteria 1976), and in the United States (Salber 1966).

The data from the populations in Table 2.1 and the subpopulations in Guatemala, Taiwan, Senegal, the Philippines, and the United States are plotted in Figure 2.2. To summarize this relationship between breastfeeding and amenorrhea a number of curves were fitted; the best fit was provided by:

$$A = 1.753e^{0.1396 \times B - 0.001872 \times B^2} \qquad R^2 = 0.96 \qquad (1)$$

A = mean or median duration of postpartum amenorrhea, in months
B = mean or median duration of breastfeeding, in months

The high correlation between the average durations of breastfeeding and amenorrhea of populations makes it possible to use this regression equation

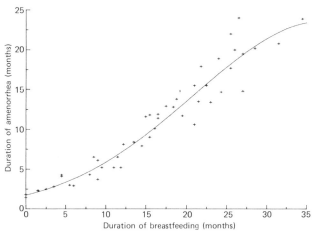

FIGURE 2.2. Mean (or median) duration of postpartum amenorrhea by duration of breastfeeding.

Table 2.1
DURATIONS OF BREASTFEEDING AND AMENORRHEA IN SELECTED POPULATIONS[a]

	Mean (median)[b] duration of breastfeeding	Mean (median)[b] duration of amenorrhea
I. U.S. (Boston)	1.5	2.3
Colombia and Venezuela (cities)	6.0	2.9
Thailand (cities)	8.0	4.3
Turkey (cities)	9.0	3.7
Egypt (cities)	11.0	5.2
Philippines (rural)	11.9	5.2
Nigeria (Lagos)	12.2	8.1
Zaire (Bukavu)	15.5	9.0
Taiwan	16.1	10.1
India (Bombay)	16.5	11.9
Senegal (Pikine)	18.4	12.8
Zaire (Ngweshe)	18.8	13.8
Guatemala (rural)	19.2	14.8
India (Khanna)	21.0	10.6
Zaire (Idjiwi)	21.8	17.9
Korea	23.0	13.5
Bangladesh (Matlab)	24.0	18.9
Senegal (rural)	24.3	14.7
Zaire (rural)	26.0	20.0
Indonesia (Mojolama)	26.5	24.0
II. Taiwan	0.0	1.8
	1-6	2.8
	7-12	5.2
	13-18	11.8
	19-24	13.5
	25+	14.8

[a] From: Lesthaeghe and Page (1980), Masnick (1979), Van Ginneken (1978).

[b] Estimates of means and medians have been combined because there is apparently little systematic difference between them, except perhaps at the shortest durations. Women who did not initiate breastfeeding (a small or negligible proportion in populations with long breastfeeding) were excluded except in Boston, Lagos, Bukavu, rural Guatemala, Senegal and Zaire, and Indonesia. Estimates taken from Lesthaeghe and Page (1980) are corrected for misreporting.

to estimate an approximate duration of amenorrhea in a population for which only breastfeeding data are available. As is evident from Figure 2.2, estimates of A obtained from the regression equation can be as much as a few months higher or lower than the "true" values, but it should be noted that at

least part of this discrepancy is due to recall, sampling, or other measurement errors in the duration of breastfeeding or amenorrhea, especially if
these data are obtained from retrospective surveys.

For individual women, the ovulation- and menstruation-inhibiting effect of
breastfeeding is somewhat less predictable than on the population level. This
is the consequence of the fact that amenorrhea is affected not only by the
duration of breastfeeding but also, and perhaps more importantly, by the
type and intensity of breastfeeding. It has been demonstrated that women
who give their infants only breast milk have a much lower probability of
resuming menstruation than women who supplement the diets of their infants
with fluids by bottle or with solid food (Huffman, Chowdhury, Chakraborty,
and Mosley 1978, McKeown and Gibson 1954, Malkani and Mirchandani
1960, Perez 1971). Many existing studies do not make a distinction between
full and partial breastfeeding and only measure the total duration of
breastfeeding, thus revealing nothing about the important changes in type
and intensity of breastfeeding that take place as the infant grows up.
Breastfeeding mothers usually give little or no other food to their infants
during the first weeks after birth. Supplemental foods are introduced slowly,
increasing in quantity over time, as the amount of breast milk demanded by
the infant reduces. The timing of the decrease in the mother's milk production is probably the principal determinant of the onset of menstruation. The
end of amenorrhea occurs frequently while the woman is still breastfeeding.
This is demonstrated in Figure 2.2 where the average duration of amenorrhea
is substantially shorter than the duration of breastfeeding. The correlation
between breastfeeding and amenorrhea is, therefore, in most women not due
to the direct effect of the termination of breastfeeding but instead is due to
the correlation between the intensity of breastfeeding in the early months
and its overall duration. In other words, populations with the longest total
durations of breastfeeding tend to have the longest periods of intense
breastfeeding that cause prolonged amenorrhea.

A number of recent investigations have clarified the physiological mechanism through which breastfeeding influences ovulation (Delvoye 1976, Konner and Worthman 1980, McNeilly 1978, Short 1976, Tyson and Perez 1978).
Although many details remain to be specified, the principal factors involved
appear to be the following. The suckling by the infant stimulates receptors in
the breast nipple that initiate a neural signal to the hypothalamus, a nerve
center in the brain. In response, the hypothalamus signals the pituitary gland
to increase the production of the hormone prolactin. Prolactin, in turn, inhibits ovulation, either by reducing the release of gonadotropic hormones
needed for ovulation or by directly affecting the ovaries. This physiological
process identifies frequent nipple stimulation as the critical factor in maintaining anovulation. Only frequent suckling as during full breastfeeding
produces a high concentration of prolactin. As the frequency and intensity of
breastfeeding decrease, average prolactin levels decline and once they fall

below a certain threshold (which possibly varies among women) ovulation resumes.

Waiting Time to Conception and Fecundability (in the Absence of Contraception)

In the following discussion, the term *conception* will refer to recognizable conceptions as is usually done in the demographic literature. Only pregnancies recognizable by the delay of the first menses after fertilization will be included, and fertilized ova that fail to implant or abort spontaneously before the woman knows she is pregnant will not be counted as conceptions.

Noncontracepting fecundable women who engage in regular intercourse take an average of several months to conceive. The most reliable and consistent estimates of the waiting time to conception are available from measurements of the interval from marriage to first birth or to first conception. Table 2.2 presents averages of these intervals for a number of populations (after exclusion of premarital conceptions). In the historical populations, the conception wait is estimated by subtracting 9 months for a full gestation and 2 months for time lost due to intrauterine mortality[1] from the interval between marriage and first birth. In the other populations, direct information about the time of the first conception after marriage was obtained, but it is likely that the waiting time to conception is slightly overestimated due to unreported fetal losses or contraceptive use. The data in Table 2.2 suggest average conception waits ranging afrom about 5 to 10 months with typical values near 7 months. This generalization applies to women in their twenties; waiting times tend to be longer for younger women in the years immediately following menarche (Balakrishnan 1979, Jain 1969), presumably because the incidence of anovulatory cycles is then higher. Conception waits are also longer among women who experience prolonged periods of separation from their spouses (for example, due to seasonal migration for work or long visits by the wife to her parental home).[2]

The duration of the waiting time to conception is determined by the rate of conception. The most widely used measure of the conception rate is *fecun-*

---

[1] The average time added to a birth interval due to intrauterine mortality is estimated by $aI/(1 - a)$, where a is the proportion of conceptions ending in an intrauterine death and I is the sum of the means of the aborted gestation, the postabortum anovulation interval, and the waiting time to conception following the spontaneous abortion (Bongaarts, 1976). With a between 0.15 and 0.20 and I around 10 months, the mean time added is about 2 months.

[2] For example, in Bangladesh the mean waiting time to conception increased from 8.6 to 11.8 and 15.3 months for corresponding durations of husband's absence of 0–1, 1–4, and 5+ months. (Pregnancies of all orders are included in these estimates.) The mean waiting time to conception for all women combined was 10.9 months (Chowdhury 1978). These estimates contain some upward bias because the conception waits of a proportion of the women overlapped with the 1974–1975 famine.

Table 2.2

OBSERVED AND ESTIMATED MEAN CONCEPTION WAITS AND FECUNDABILITIES IN THE FIRST PREGNANCY INTERVAL OF NONCONTRACEPTING WOMEN IN SELECTED POPULATIONS AND GROUPS OF POPULATIONS[a]

	Average (and range) of mean intervals between marriage and first birth, in months	Average (and range) of mean waiting times to conception before first pregnancy, in months	Average (and range) of estimated mean fecundabilities in first pregnancy interval
Historical populations			
15 English parishes	19.0 (17.3 – 20.8)	8.0 (6.3 – 9.8)[c]	.22 (.18 – .25)
13 German villages	17.9 (16.4 – 19.5)	6.9 (5.4 – 8.5)[c]	.23 (.18 – .26)
2 Belgian communities	17.0 (16.7 – 17.3)	6.0 (5.7 – 6.3)[c]	.28 (.28 – .29)
3 French communities	17.0 (16.3 – 17.3)	6.0 (5.3 – 6.3)[c]	.23 (.18 – .31)
Developing countries [b]			
4 Latin American countries	—	7.9 (6.7 – 8.9)	.18 (.16 – .21)
Taiwan	—	6.3	.22
Other populations			
U.S. (PFS)	—	10.0	.18
Hutterites	—	4.7	.25

a/ From: Balakrishnan (1979), Bongaarts (1975), Jain (1969a), Leridon (1977), Majumdar and Sheps (1970), Potter and Parker (1964), Westoff, Potter, Sagi and Mishler (1961), Wilson (1980).

b/ Women aged 20–24

c/ Estimated, see text.

dability, defined as the probability of conceiving in a month among fecundable women (i.e., pregnant, sterile, and amenorrheic women are excluded, Gini 1924). Estimates of levels of fecundability following marriage are also presented in Table 2.2. A fairly typical value for fecundability appears to be 0.2, which means that, in a group of fecundable women, 20% can be expected to conceive in the first month of exposure to the risk of conception. Fecundability is inversely related to the duration of the conception wait; the higher fecundability, the shorter the conception wait, and vice versa. In fact it can be shown that there is an exact inverse relationship between the conception wait, W, and fecundability f: $W = 1/f$, in a homogeneous population of women with identical levels of fecundability (Henry 1953, Sheps and Menken 1973). However, in reality fecundability is not the same for all women because they have different frequencies of intercourse and different biological characteristics. In such a heterogeneous population the average waiting time to conception is longer than in the homogeneous case, as with heterogeneity women with the highest fecundability conceive quickest, leaving slower conceivers with decreasing levels of fecundability in successive months (Potter and Parker 1964). In the populations in Table 2.2, the observed waiting time to conception is on the average about 50% longer than the inverse of fecundability, so that an approximate estimate of W is provided by the equation $W = 1.5/f$.

The estimates of the waiting time to conception and fecundability in Table 2.2 are for the period immediately after marriage for women mostly in their twenties, the prime childbearing years. As frequency of intercourse tends to decline with age and/or duration of marriage, one can expect a rise in the average conception wait as women grow older. (It should be noted that with increasing age the distributions of conception delays becomes more skewed. The mean is therefore not always a satisfactory indicator, but there are no readily available alternatives). Unfortunately, the available data are insufficient to make reliable generalizations about the extent of this rise. Taiwan is the only population in which estimates of the conception wait before the first pregnancy can be compared with the wait before later pregnancies. The former averages 6.3 months (see Table 2.2) and the latter about 6.8 months (obtained by subtracting the 10.1-month postpartum amenorrhea interval from the 16.9-month interpregnancy interval after a live birth, Jain 1969). This suggests that the change in the waiting time to conception for successive birth intervals may be modest, at least for ages up to the late thirties. Supporting this tentative conclusion are two other findings. First, observed increases with age in average closed-birth intervals in natural fertility populations are quite small; increases in different populations range from 10 to 25% between age groups 20–24 and 35–39[3] (Henry 1953, Potter, Wyon, Parker,

---

[3] The observed change with age in the average birth interval depends on whether age is measured at the beginning or at the end of the birth intervals. The former introduces a negative bias in the older age groups due to the truncating effect of the onset of sterility, and the latter is

and Gordon 1965). If the average birth interval changes little with increasing age, then the birth interval components such as the conception wait for the post-partum amenorrhea interval can only lengthen by relatively modest amounts. Second, a comparison of the mean interval between marriage and first birth with the mean of birth intervals in which the infant died shortly after birth indicates little difference in the conception wait between these two intervals. The latter should be 1.5 or 2 months longer than the former (to allow for a minimum amenorrhea interval) in case the conception waits are the same. This has indeed been observed. For example, in 13 German villages studied by Knodel (1979) the mean birth interval was 19.7 months if the infant died within a month after birth and the average interval from marriage to first birth was 17.9 months (Wilson 1980).

One of the most striking aspects of the conception data presented here is that only about one in five noncontracepting women conceives in a month despite engaging in regular intercourse and that the time to conceive can easily exceed 6 months. These conception rates are lower than one might have expected a priori. An explanation for these findings will be provided next.

Fecundability and the Frequency of Intercourse

The fecundability of a population is directly dependent on the frequency of intercourse. This is demonstrated in a unique study by Barrett and Marshall (1969) who analyzed daily calendars with information on the timing of intercourse and ovulation in a group of 241 noncontracepting British women of proven fertility. From these records the fecundabilities of women with dif-

---

associated with a negative bias at younger ages because shorter intervals have a higher chance of ending at an early age (Potter, Wyon, Parker, and Gordon 1965, Sheps and Menken 1973). In addition, there is possibly a small upward bias in the oldest age groups, if age is measured at the end of the birth interval, as longer birth intervals have a better chance of ending at a higher age. To solve this problem, Potter, Wyon, Parker, and Gordon (1965) suggest that a reasonable trend with age is obtained by using birth intervals that start in age groups 20–24 and 25–29 in combination with birth intervals that end in the older age groups. With this method, Potter, Wyon, Parker, and Gordon (1965) found a rise in the birth interval from 30.1 months in age group 20–24 to 35.8 in age group 35–39 in a study in India. This increase of 5.7 months or 19% is attributable to five factors: (a) an increase in intrauterine mortality; (b) a lengthening of the waiting time to conception and a decline in fecundability associated with decreasing frequency of intercourse and/or a rise in undetected embryonic mortality; (c) a lengthening of the postpartum amenorrhea interval; (d) the use of some contraception presumably to a greater extent among older women; and (e) the small upward bias in the estimates of mean birth intervals at older ages. Another indication of the generally small rise in birth intervals with age is given by the modest decline with age in the fertility of fecund women, which is inversely related to the mean birth interval in natural fertility populations. In historical populations, the fecund fertility rate in the age group 35–39 is typically between 10 and 25% lower than in the age group 20–24 (Charbonneaux 1979, Henry 1961).

ferent frequencies of intercourse in the 6-day period around the time of ovulation were calculated by dividing the number of conception cycles by the total number of cycles observed in each group:

Number of coital acts in 6-day period	Observed fecundability
1	0.17 (=33/192)
2	0.34 (=27/80)
3	0.41 (=19/46)
4	0.38 (= 5/13)

Although these results are subject to large sampling errors, there is a strong positive effect of coital frequency on fecundability. To understand this relationship, it is necessary to examine the biological factors involved in the conception process.

A recognizable conception takes place during a given menstrual cycle only if (a) the cycle is ovulatory; (b) insemination occurs during the fertile period in the middle of the cycle; (c) insemination during the fertile period leads to a fertilization; and (d) fertilization results in a recognizable conception (James 1979, Potter 1961). If the probabilities of these four events are denoted by the variables $p1, p2, p3$, and $p4$, respectively, then the fecundability, f, is simply equal to their product: $f = p1 \times p2 \times p3 \times p4$.

$p1$

The probability that a cycle is anovulatory is fairly small, except in the years immediately following menarche or preceding menopause. Based on evidence from a number of studies, Potter (1961) estimates the incidence of anovulatory cycles in the central childbearing years at about 5%, so that $p1$ = 0.95. Investigations have attempted to measure the incidence of anovulation from the presence or absence of a shift in the basal body temperature (BBT) in midcycle, but this BBT method is not entirely reliable (Moghissi, 1980).

$p2$

Conception is possible only during the so-called fertile period, a brief interval around the time of ovulation. As will be shown in the next section, the duration of the fertile period is about 2 days. The probability of having at least one coitus coincide with a fertile period of 2 days is given by the following equation:

$$p2 = 1 - (M - n)(M - n - 1)/(M^2 - M) \qquad (2)$$

where n is the number of coital acts occurring during an interval of M days (e.g., a month or a week) that includes the fertile period (this equation is directly derived from a more general model proposed by Glass and Grebenik 1954). It is assumed that intercourse takes place at random during the interval M, with at most one coitus per day.

$p3$

Even in case a coitus coincides with the fertile period of an ovulatory cycle, a fertilization does not always follow. Several things can go wrong (for example, the sperm may be low in quality or the ovum incapable of fertilization, and either the sperm or ovum could fail to reach the fallopian tubes). Although little is known about these possible unfavorable outcomes, they are generally considered to occur infrequently (Hertig 1967, James 1979). We will assume $p3 = 0.95$, which is slightly higher than the estimate of Hertig (1967).[4]

$p4$

Hertig (1967) estimated that only half of the fertilized ova yield a recognizable conception so that $p4 = 0.5$. The remainder either fail to implant or abort spontaneously before the first missed menses.

Multiplying the probabilities $p1-p4$ gives the following estimate of fecundability for women in the central childbearing years:

$$f = p1 \times p2 \times p3 \times p4 = 0.45 (1 - (M - n)$$
$$(M - n - 1)/(M^2 - M)) \quad (3)$$

Model estimates of f for different coital rates n can now be made if M is specified. Because the average duration of the menstrual cycle equals about 29 days (Treloar, Boynton, Behn, and Brown, 1967, Vollman 1956), one can estimate the average intermenstruum interval during which virtually all intercourse takes place at about 26 days. With $M = 26$, Equation (3) yields the estimates of fecundability presented in Table 2.3. As the number of coital acts increases from 1 to 20 per cycle, fecundability rises from 0.035 to 0.429. The relationship is not linear; the increments in fecundability become smaller as coital frequency rises.

Strictly speaking, Equation (3) should only be applied in a homogeneous population. In the heterogeneous case, substitution of the *average* number of

[4] Hertig (1967) estimates that fertilization did not occur in 15% of a group of women who had intercourse within 24 hr before or after the time of ovulation as determined from the endometrial morphology. If all these women had intercourse during the fertile period, $p3$ would be 0.85, but this is likely to be an underestimate. Some women probably missed the fertile period, partly because the time of ovulation cannot be determined with complete accuracy and partly because the fertile period does not extend to 24 hr past the time of ovulation (see text).

Table 2.3
MODEL ESTIMATES OF FECUNDABILITY AND CONCEPTION WAIT FOR DIFFERENT
COITAL RATES

Number of coital acts per menstrual cycle [a]	Average coital frequency per week	Fecundability	Approximate duration of conception wait [b] (in months)
1	.27	.035	42.8
2	.54	.068	22.1
3	.81	.100	15.0
4	1.08	.130	11.5
5	1.35	.159	9.4
6	1.62	.187	8.0
7	1.88	.213	7.0
8	2.15	.238	6.3
9	2.42	.262	5.7
10	2.69	.284	5.3
11	2.96	.305	4.9
12	3.23	.324	4.6
13	3.50	.342	4.4
14	3.77	.359	4.2
15	4.04	.374	4.0
20	5.38	.429	3.5

[a] All coital acts are assumed to take place during the intermenstruum
interval with an estimated average duration of 26 days.

[b] Estimated as $1.5/f$, see text.

coital acts per cycle in the equation yields a slight overestimate of fecundability.[5] However, Equation (3) calculates fecundability per cycle, and, if an
estimate per month is required, a correction is required because the average
month is longer than the average menstrual cycle. Fortunately, these two
relatively small errors nearly compensate one another, and the results in
Table 2.3 derived from Equation (3) can therefore be accepted as estimates
of fecundability per month in a heterogeneous population.

[5] A formula for estimating the correction factor required in the heterogeneous case is given in
Bongaarts (1976). The size of the correction varies with the mean and variance of the coital rate
distribution, but a typical correction is around 5%.

The last column of Table 2.3 presents the approximate average duration of the conception wait (estimated at $1.5/f$) for the different levels of coital frequency. The results indicate that the normal range of 5–10 months for the average conception wait is associated with coital rates between 4 and 11 per intermenstruum or between 1.25 and 2.9 per week. Coital rates reported by women in their twenties in a variety of populations fall within this range (Cartwright 1976, Leridon 1977, Nag 1972, Ware 1979, Westoff 1974) thus giving a very crude indication of plausibility of the results in Table 2.3.

The validity of Equation (3) can be tested directly by comparing its estimates of fecundability for different coital rates with the levels observed in the study by Barrett and Marshall. Substituting $M = 6$ and $n = 1, 2, 3$, and 4, in Equation (3) and setting $p1 = 1.0$ because anovulatory cycles were excluded yields fecundability estimates of 0.16, 0.29, 0.38 and 0.44, respectively. These model estimates agree quite well with the observed values 0.17, 0.34, 0.41, and 0.39. This suggests that the biological mechanism linking coital frequency and fecundability outlined here is fairly realistic.

The relationship between coital frequency and fecundability presented here is basically a revised version of an equation originally proposed by Glass and Grebenik (1954). Alternative models have been proposed by Barrett and Marshall (1969) and Schwartz MacDonald and Henchel (1980), but these studies assume a duration of the fertile period of about a week. As will be demonstrated next, this assumption is probably not realistic.

The Probability of Conception on Different Days of the Menstrual Cycle

The exact duration of the fertile period has proven difficult to determine, and, as a consequence, the existing estimates vary widely—from less than a day (Tietze 1960) to a week or more (Hartman 1962). The basic biological and demographic data available for determining the duration of the fertile period will be discussed briefly first, before the principal cause of the divergence in estimates can be identified.

THE BIOLOGICAL EVIDENCE

The fertile period is a brief interval around the time of ovulation during which an insemination can result in a fertilization. Fertilization is possible if insemination occurs before ovulation because sperm retains its fertility for a short time after insemination. Fertilization can also take place following ovulation because the ovum remains viable for a brief interval. An approximate estimate of the fertile period therefore would be the sum of the fertile life times of sperm and ovum, but this estimate is slightly too high because it does not take into account the time required for sperm capacitation. Sperm needs about 6 hr after insemination before becoming fertile (Gwatkin 1977,

James 1979) and this time should be subtracted to yield an accurate estimate
of the fertile period:

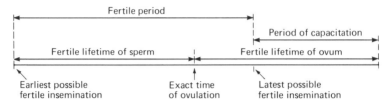

Best available estimates of the fertile life times range from 24 to 48 hr for
sperm (Vander Vliet and Hafez 1974) and from 12 to 24 hr for the ovum
(Barrett and Marshall 1969). Summing these life times and subtracting 6 hr
for capacitation gives a range of 30–66 hr for the fertile period with an
average of about 48 hr or 2 days.

Although fertilization is only possible during the fertile period, a fertilization or a (recognizable) conception does not always follow an insemination
during the fertile period. The probability that fertilization during the fertile
period fails is about 5% ($p3$ = 0.95) and the probability of a recognizable
conception is 0.475 ($p3 \times p4$ = 0.95 × 0.5). Based on these estimates, the
probability of conceiving around the time of ovulation is plotted in Figure
2.3a. The risk of conception is 0 until the beginning of the fertile period. It
then rises to 0.475, and, after about 2 days, it declines again to 0. The
"shape" of the fertile period is approximately rectangular according to this
biological model.

THE DEMOGRAPHIC EVIDENCE

A few studies have attempted to measure directly the probability of conceiving on days around the approximate time of ovulation. Vollman (1953),
for example, analyzed calendars with daily records of the occurrence of
intercourse in a group of noncontracepting women. The probability of conception on different days before and after the fourteenth day of the cycle can
be calculated from these records. The results are plotted in Figure 2.3c. The
probability of conceiving is virtually 0 before the eighth and after the
twenty-third day of the menstrual cycle, and it reaches a maximum of less
than 0.1 in the middle of the cycle.[6] Assuming an average incidence of
anovulatory cycles among the women in this study, the daily probabilities of
conception among ovulating women would be about 5% higher.

A similar set of data was available to Barrett and Marshall (1969). In
addition to daily intercourse records, they collected daily temperature charts
from which the approximate time of ovulation can be determined by the
temperature shift (BBT method). From the menstrual cycles in which only

[6] Three conceptions occurring 28, 29, and 36 days after the onset of the last menstrual period
are excluded. It may be assumed that recording errors were made or that the cycles were
abnormal.

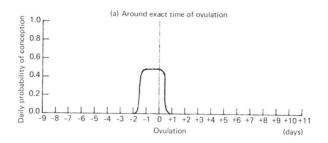

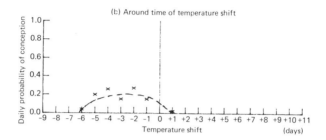

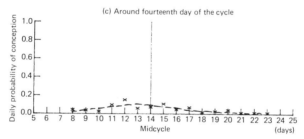

FIGURE 2.3. Daily probabilities of conception around exact or approximate time of ovulation (x = observed. ___ = estimated. --- = smoothed).

one coitus took place in a 7-day period around the time of the temperature shift, the following daily conception probabilities can be calculated (Schwartz, Macdonald, and Henchel 1980, p. 399):

	Time of intercourse	Observed fecundability
Days before temperature shift	−6	0.04
	−5	0.20
	−4	0.26
	−3	0.15
	−2	0.27
	−1	0.15
Days after temperature shift	+1	0.07

These results are plotted in Figure 2.3b. The fertile period ranged from 6 days before to 1 day after the temperature shift, and the conception risk reached a maximum of about .25 a few days before the shift.

How can one explain these apparently large discrepancies between the different approaches to the estimation of the fertile period? As is shown in Figure 2.3, the demographic studies yield much longer fertile periods and lower conception risks than the biological model. Fortunately there is a simple explanation. The demographic studies can be shown to be in good agreement with the biological model if account is taken of the fact that neither the fourteenth day of a cycle nor the day of the temperature shift gives the exact timing of ovulation. That the middle of the menstrual cycle is not a good indicator of the time of ovulation is well known (Hartman 1962) but the BBT method also yields errors of up to several days[7] (Buxton and Engle 1950, Hartman 1962, James 1969, Vollmann 1953). As a result, the curves in Figure 2.3b and 2.3c represent average conception rates of women whose fertile periods start at different points in time. In other words, the approximately rectangular shape of the fertile period is "spread out" in the demographic studies as Figure 2.3 indicates. This distortion of the true shape is largest in Figure 2.3c because the fourteenth day of the cycle is a less accurate indicator of ovulation than the temperature shift. If this hypothesis is correct, then the areas under the three curves in Figure 2.3 should be equal. Actually, the areas for Figures 2.3a, b, and c are 0.95 (= 2 × 0.475), 1.14, and 0.88, respectively. The agreement is quite good considering the various assumptions made in the biological model and the sampling errors in the demographic studies. It can therefore be concluded that the demographic results are consistent with an approximately rectangular fertile period of about 2 days duration. This conclusion is supported by realistic relationships between the frequency of intercourse and fecundability found in the preceding section where the fertile period was assumed to equal 2 days. (In reality the fertile period is unlikely to be exactly rectangular, but, as shown by Potter 1961, even a trapezoidal shape with the same average duration would give virtually the same estimates of fecundability for a given frequency of intercourse.)

Spontaneous Intrauterine Mortality

Measures of intrauterine mortality usually include both spontaneous abortions and stillbirths, but exclude embryonic deaths before the first missed

---

[7] In addition to a random error, there appears to be a systematic error. The temperature shift occurs on average about 2 days after the actual time of ovulation. Vollman (1953) reports that the temperature shift follows by about 2 days the "mittelschmertz," an intermenstrual pain believed to be associated with the rupture of the ovarian follicle.

menses. A *spontaneous abortion* is a fetal death before the twenty-eighth week of gestation. After that date the fetus becomes viable and a fetal death is called a *stillbirth*. The duration of gestation is customarily measured from the first day of the last menstrual period and is about 2 weeks longer than the true duration of pregnancy.

A substantial number of studies have attempted to estimate the risk of intrauterine mortality but they often suffer from significant shortcomings (Leridon 1977, WHO 1970a). Among the problems encountered are (*a*) incomplete reporting of fetal deaths, especially of early spontaneous abortions in retrospective studies; (*b*) unrepresentative nature of the study population; (*c*) overstatement of spontaneous fetal mortality due to inclusion of induced abortions or misreporting of delayed menses; (*d*) errors in statistical estimation procedures; and (*d*) sampling errors if only a small number of fetal death are observed. As a consequence, only a few studies can be considered reliable.

Excluding retrospective studies and others with obvious deficiencies, leaves four reports, all in the United States, with presumably reliable estimates of intrauterine mortality by duration of gestation.[8] In these four studies (Erhardt 1963, French and Bierman 1962, Shapiro, Levine, and Abramowitz 1970, Taylor 1970), the average risk of an intrauterine death per 100 pregnancies in progress at 4 weeks from the last menstrual period is:

Gestational age (weeks)	Intrauterine mortality (%)
4–7	8.1
8–11	5.9
12–15	2.9
16–19	1.0
20–23	0.6
24–27	0.3
28–31	0.2
32–36	0.2
36–39	0.3
40+	0.5
	Total 20.0

[8] Leridon (1977) examined seven studies that give lifetable estimates of intrauterine mortality. From these seven, the Petterson study is excluded here because no fetal deaths after the twenty-fourth week were observed. Only one of the three lifetables from Shapiro's work is selected here because in one case (Shapiro, Jones and Densen 1962) the fetal mortality in the 4–8-week period is obviously underestimated and, in another, the estimates of intrauterine mortality are biased upward (Shapiro, Levine, and Abramowitz 1970).

The overall risk of an intrauterine death after the fourth gestational week is about 20% (as noted earlier, the risk is much higher before the fourth week). The risk declines steeply from a high of 8.1% in the second month of gestation to a low of 0.2% around the eighth month, rising slightly thereafter. The large majority of deaths occur early in gestation. The risk of fetal mortality in the period from 4 to 8 weeks is likely to be slightly overestimated, because in a number of cases a conception and fetal death were recorded solely on the basis of a report of a delayed menstruation. The actual proportion of conceptions failing to yield a live birth is therefore probably slightly smaller, say around 17%. It is in practice very difficult to determine with certainty whether a fetal death takes place before the fifth or sixth week of gestation, except if a positive pregnancy test has been obtained. Menstrual delays of over a week occur not infrequently among nonpregnant women (Treloar, Boynton, Behn, and Brown 1967) and widely used pregnancy tests are not very reliable during the first 2 weeks after the missed menses (Miller, Fortney, and Kessel 1976). It would therefore be preferable to estimate intrauterine mortality from the sixth week of gestation when pregnancies can be reliably established, but most existing studies group estimates in the standard 4-week periods. Presumably, the risk of fetal death after 6 weeks would be near 15%.

Intrauterine mortality rates vary substantially with age. They are lowest in the early twenties, rising slowly to the mid-thirties, and increasing sharply thereafter. Women aged 40–44 experience fetal mortality at about double the average rate. Teeenagers may also have higher rates than women in their twenties, but this is not consistently observed (Leridon 1977, Nortman 1974).

Although very limited, the available evidence suggests that differences in intrauterine mortality between developing and developed countries may be quite small. Several carefully designed retrospective studies have been conducted in developing countries and they report fetal mortality rates in the same 12–15% range found in retrospective studies in developed countries (Leridon 1977). In addition, there is one reliable prospective study in Pakistan that estimates intrauterine mortality at 17.6% after the sixth gestational week (Awan 1974). This estimate is close to the levels observed in the United States. Another prospective investigation in Bangladesh (Chen, Ahmed, Gesche, and Mosley 1974) reports an overall fetal death rate of 14.9, but it is based on a small sample, including only 14 fetal deaths. Further research is required before one can accept the hypothesis that intrauterine mortality is relatively invariant among populations, but this hypothesis is broadly consistent with current understanding of the etiology of intrauterine mortality. In the early months of gestation, the majority of fetal deaths are caused by genetic defects (Leridon 1977, WHO 1970a) although other biological factors such as ectopic pregnancies also play a role. As these biological causes presumably operate relatively independently from social, economic, and health factors (except for a few specific diseases), one can expect relatively little variation in early fetal mortality that constitutes the bulk of all intrauterine mortality. In the later months of pregnancy, the fetus becomes more susceptible to such factors as infections and the general health of the mother (Yerushalmy, Bierman, Kemp, Conner, and French 1955). Stillbirth rates are indeed higher by about 3% in poor developing countries (WHO 1970b), but this has a relatively small effect on the overall intrauterine mortality rate.

Prevalence of Permanent Sterility

Menopause signals the definite end of the potential reproductive years of women. In developed countries the mean age at menopause ranges from about 47 to 50 years (medians slightly higher) (Gray 1979a, McMahon and Worcester 1966). The few estimates in developing countries are much less consistent, ranging from 43.7 to 50.7 years (Bongaarts 1980). The quality of some of these estimates is questionable, and errors due to age misreporting, inaccurate recall, or inappropriate statistical analysis account for at least part of the variation (Gray, 1979a, McKinley, Jefferys, and Thompson 1972, MacMahon and Worcester 1966). It is therefore not clear whether there is a systematic difference in the mean age at menopause between developing and developed countries. If such a difference exists, it is probably rather small.

Sterility or *infecundity* is defined as the physiological incapacity to produce a live birth. Although a woman can be certain that she is sterile after menopause, actual sterility or severe subfecundity may set in years earlier. Several causes can be identified:

1. A number of abnormalities of the reproductive system that prevent otherwise healthy women from conceiving and bearing offspring even during the prime-childbearing years (Speroff, Glass, and Kase 1978)

2. a high incidence of irregular and anovulatory cycles in the years immediately preceding menopause (Gray 1979b, Metcalf 1979, Treloar 1967)

3. A rapid rise in intrauterine mortality and undetected embryonic mortality among women in their forties (Gray 1979b)

4. A high prevalence of specific diseases, primarily gonorrhea and genital tuberculosis (Gray 1979a).

The first three factors affect all populations probably to a similar extent; the impact of the fourth factor varies widely, from highly significant in some African societies (Belsey 1976, Gray 1979a, Retel-Laurentin 1979, Romaniuk 1968) to small or absent in most other populations. In addition to female sterility, there is of course sterility of the male, which is the cause of couple sterility in a third to a half of all cases (McFalls 1979, Troen and Oshima 1980). The best available estimates of couple sterility have been calculated from historical data by Henry (1965) who developed a special methodology for this purpose[9]. He estimates the following proportions of sterility among couples by age of the wife:

Age of wife	Percentage of sterile couples
20	3
25	5
30	8
35	15
40	32
45	(69)[10]
50	100

About 3% of couples are sterile from the beginning of the reproductive period and will consequently remain childless. Similar levels of childlessness are observed in developing countries with high fertility (Conception 1981). With increasing age, the sterile proportion rises, slowly until the late thirties and rapidly thereafter, reaching 100% at age 50. Comparable data for contemporary developed countries are not available, partly because the methodology developed by Henry requires that natural fertility prevails. Another complication encountered in determining the prevalence of natural sterility in developed countries is the relatively high number of sterilizing operations. For example, 30% of U.S. women aged 35–44 in 1976 underwent sterilizing operations, 17% for noncontraceptive and 13% for contraceptive reasons (Ford 1978).

The mean age at onset of sterility can be estimated at 41.7 years, based on the age-specific proportions sterile of Henry. This mean is well below the mean age at menopause for reasons already given. If the onset of sterility occurs on the average in the early forties, then the end of childbearing in populations with natural fertility should take place at an even earlier age because sterile women cannot be fertile, but fecund women can be infertile at least for brief periods. The end of childbearing or the onset of infertility is measured by the mean age at last birth. Table 2.4 summarizes data on the mean age at last birth for a number of populations with natural fertility. The average of these estimates is 40 years, which, as expected, is slightly below

[9] Henry (1965) estimates the proportion fecund in an age group by dividing the fertility rate of all married women by the fertility rate of married women who are fecund. The latter is estimated as the fertility rate of married women who have a birth after the upper limit of the age group (e.g., after age 34 for age group 30–34). This method is only accurate up to age 40 and in populations with natural fertility.

[10] Henry (1965) does not give an estimate of sterility for age 45 because he considers his methodology unreliable at that age. The estimate given here is taken from Vincent (1950), who proposed a set age-specific sterility proportion almost identical to Henry's.

Table 2.4

ESTIMATES OF THE MEAN AGE AT LAST BIRTH IN HISTORICAL POPULATIONS[a]

German villages (pre-1850)	
Grafenhausen	39.7
Oshselbronn	39.2
Three Bavarian villages	40.6
Four Waldeck villages	40.7
Werdum	39.4
All villages	
Age at marriage: 25	40.3
25–29	40.1
Occupation of husband: Artisans, etc.	39.8
Farmers	39.8
Landless	40.1
Number of infant deaths in first	
two confinements: 0	40.1
1	40.4
2	40.4
North American communities	
Canada (seventeenth century)	40.1
Canada (eighteenth century)	41.0
Bois-Vert	40.7
St. Jean-de-Cherbourg	38.6
Hingham	39.1
Quakers	39.6
Hutterites	40.9
Bris	38.7
French parishes	
Crulai	40.0
Tourouvre au Perche	40.3
English population (mid-nineteenth century)	41.7

[a] From Charbonneaux (1970, 1979), Frisch (1978), Gautier and Henry (1958), and Knodel (1978).

the mean age at onset of sterility. The data in Table 2.4 indicate that the mean age at last birth is remarkably invariant. With few exceptions the means fall in the 39–41 year range even when subpopulations with different ages at marriage, occupations of husband, and numbers of infant deaths are considered. It would be unrealistic to expect all populations to be in this narrow range because factors such as taboos against intercourse at older ages (Caldwell and Caldwell 1977, Ware 1979), disease-induced sterility, and age misreporting can cause the actual or observed mean age to be lower. Nevertheless, the uniformity of estimates in Table 2.4 and the fact that the well-nourished and healthy Hutterite population has a mean age at last birth of 40.9 suggest that the timing of the onset of natural sterility varies little among populations, except in cases where gonorrhea or genital tuberculosis is widespread.

THE EFFECT OF THE PROXIMATE DETERMINANTS ON
NATURAL FERTILITY

Although all five proximate determinants can affect natural fertility, their impact differs substantially, and in practice most variation in natural fertility is due to variations in just two or three of the proximate determinants. To identify these most important proximate determinants, we will go through an arithmetical exercise (a so-called sensitivity analysis) consisting of three steps. First, a simple reproductive model will be described that estimates the total fertility rate in a hypothetical natural fertility population if estimates of the five proximate determinants are available. Next, each of the proximate determinants is varied through its normal observed range while the other determinants are left constant at a standard level, and the corresponding change in natural fertility is noted. Finally, a ranking of the sizes of the variations in natural fertility caused by the changes in each of the proximate determinants yields a ranking of their importance in causing variations in natural fertility.

The basic segmentation of the childbearing years into birth intervals and birth interval components used in this model exercise is summarized in Figure 1.1 (see p. 4). The *total fertility rate* is estimated as the number of birth intervals between marriage and the end of the childbearing years, and the *birth interval* equals the sum of its components (the postpartum infecundable period, the waiting time to conception, time added by intrauterine mortality, and a full-term pregnancy). For example, a population with a mean age at marriage of 22.5 years and a mean age at the end of childbearing of 40 years would have a 17.5-year childbearing span, and with a mean birth interval of 2.5 years the total fertility rate would be 7 births per woman (17.5/2.5). An average birth interval of 2.5 years could consist of (on average) 1-year postpartum infecundability, 0.6-years conception delay, 0.15 years added by intrauterine mortality, and 0.75 years for a full-term gestation.

Estimates of the approximate observed ranges of the proximate determinants in a wide variety of natural fertility populations based on the preceding review are presented in Table 2.5. These ranges cover what might be considered normal values, that is, the large majority of natural fertility populations can be expected to fall within the ranges given. Not included here are exceptional cases, such as populations in parts of tropical Africa with high levels of pathological sterility due to venereal disease. Similarly, populations in which spousal separation is exceptionally frequent or prolonged would have longer conception delays than is allowed for here. Terminal abstinence is also assumed to be negliable.

The sensitivity analysis is carried out by varying the proximate determinants through their ranges one at a time, whereas the other determinants are set at the "standard" values given in the last column of Table 2.5. These standard values together produce a total fertility rate of 7 (a 17.5-year childbearing span with 2.5-year birth intervals.) Any change in a proximate

Table 2.5

**APPROXIMATE OBSERVED RANGES AND STANDARD MODEL VALUES
OF POPULATION AVERAGES OF PROXIMATE DETERMINANTS OF
NATURAL FERTILITY**

Proximate determinants	Approximate range of averages (years)	Model standard (years)
Age at marriage	15.0 – 27.5	22.5
Age at end of childbearing years	38.5 – 41.0	40.0
Duration of postpartum infecundability	0.25 – 2.0	1.0
Conception delay	0.4 – 0.85	0.6
Time added by intrauterine mortality	0.1 – 0.2	0.15

determinant results in a departure from this standard total fertility rate of 7. The extent of the change in fertility is estimated with the simple numerical model already described. For example, an increase in postpartum infecundability interval from 1 to 2 years would change the average birth interval from 2.5 to 3.5 years and would produce only 5 births in 17.5 years of actual childbearing. The results of the complete sensitivity analysis are plotted in Figure 2.4. The largest variations in the total fertility rate are caused by changes in age at marriage and in the duration of postpartum infecundability, and the smallest fertility variations are found for the end of the childbearing years and spontaneous intrauterine mortality. (These findings should be considered approximate, because of a lack of detailed information about the

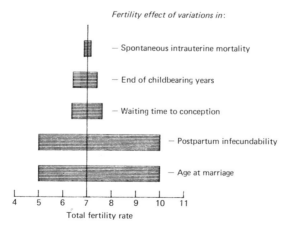

FIGURE 2.4.   Variations in the total fertility rate induced by variations in five proximate determinants of natural fertility.

distribution of the proximate variables within the ranges used here.) As age at marriage increases from 15 to 27.5 years, the total fertility rate (TFR) declines from 10 to 5. In contrast, an increase in the average time added by spontaneous intrauterine mortality from .1 to .2 years produced only a small decline in the total fertility rate, from 7.14 to 6.86. We can, therefore, conclude that variations in age at marriage and the duration of postpartum infecundability are, in general, the most important determinant of variations in natural fertility. This conclusion does not imply that marriage and postpartum infecundability are always the only or even the principal causes of differences in natural fertility. For example, the effect of variations in the conception delay, which cause the TFR to deviate 0.6 births from the standard value of 7, is quite respectable by itself, even though it is much smaller than the effects of age at marriage and postpartum infecundability.

One final comment about the standard population used here. Although the standard values of the proximate determinants are roughly in the middle of the observed ranges, as is the standard total fertility rate of 7, this standard population is not representative of any class of natural fertility populations. Contemporary developing countries with fertility close to natural levels typically have lower mean ages at marriage and longer postpartum infecundability than the standard population. As these two effects tend to compensate one another, the resulting observed total fertility rate is often still around 7 births per woman. In historical European societies, marriage is typically later than 22.5 years. The total fertility rate is therefore lower, despite some compensatory effect from a shorter postpartum infecundability interval that usually is between 6 and 12 months. Finally, in contemporary developed countries, postpartum infecundability is short because large proportions of women do not breast-feed at all or those who do so, breast-feed only a short time (Jeliffe, Jeliffe, Sai, and Senanayaka 1979, Martinez and Nalezienski 1979, WHO 1981). A postpartum infecundability interval of 3 months would, according to the model, yield a total fertility rate of 10 if no contraception and induced abortion is practiced.

SUMMARY

The foregoing review of the proximate determinants of natural marital fertility has touched only on the highlights of what has now become a large literature. It is demonstrated that the duration of postpartum amenorrhea varies widely among populations, from a few months to about 2 years, largely if not entirely as a result of differences in breastfeeding behavior. The waiting time to conception is found to vary within a narrower range, typically no more than 2 or 3 months from the average of about 7 months. Frequency of intercourse is the principal factor affecting the conception delay and fecundability. The remaining two proximate determinants, spontaneous intrauterine mortality and the prevalence of natural permanent sterility, apparently are relatively constant and are not directly influenced by behavior. Among the four proximate determinants of natural marital fertility, postpartum amenorrhea is the only one for which there is clear evidence of an important change with modernization. In most developing countries or historical populations, the duration of postpartum amenorrhea exceeds 6 months, and it is often well over a year, while in contemporary developed countries amenorrhea is usually much briefer. Although it is yet to be clearly documented, modernization might also influence sexual behavior and fecundability, but any such changes will usually have a much smaller impact on fertility than the shortening of postpartum amenorrhea.

A comparison of the changes in natural fertility induced by the different proximate determinants yielded a ranking of the importance of the proximate determinants in causing variations in natural fertility. Age at marriage and postpartum amenorrhea were found to be by far the most important determinants of natural fertility, primarily because of their wide range. For example, a change in postpartum amenorrhea from 2 years to 3 months causes fertility to double. This implies that, at least theoretically, differences in postpartum amenorrhea could explain most of the observed differences in marital fertility of populations with natural fertility. In contrast, the waiting time to conception had a much smaller impact, and normal variations in spontaneous intrauterine mortality and permanent natural sterility had only little effect on fertility, according to this analysis with a reproductive model.

REFERENCES

Awan, A. K. (1975), "Some Biological Correlates of Pregnancy Wastage," *American Journal of Obstetrics and Gynecology, 119*, 4, 525–532.

Balakrishnan, T. R. (1979), "Probability of Conception, Conception Delay and Estimates of Fecundability in Rural and Semi-urban Areas of Certain Latin American Countries," *Social Biology, 26*, 226–231.

Barrett, J. C. and J. Marshall (1969), "The Risk of Conception on Different Days of the Menstrual Cycle," *Population Studies, 23*, 3, 455–461.

Belsey, M. (1976), "The Epidemiology of Infertility: A Review with Particular Reference to Subsaharan Africa," *Bulletin of the World Health Organization, 54*.

Bongaarts, J. (1975), "A Method for the Estimation of Fecundability," *Demography, 12*, 4, 645–659.

Bongaarts, J. (1976), "Intermediate Fertility Variables and Marital Fertility Rates," *Population Studies, 30*, 2, 227–241.

Bongaarts, J. (1980), "Does Malnutrition Affect Fecundity? A Summary of Evidence," *Science, 208*, 564–569.

Bongaarts, J. and J. Menken (1982), "The Supply of Children: A Critical Essay," in *Determinants of Fertility in Developing Countries: A Summary of Knowledge*, National Academy of Sciences (forthcoming).

Buxton, C. L. and E. T. Engle (1950), "Time of Ovulation," *American Journal of Obstetrics and Gynecology, 60*, 3, 539–553.

Caldwell, J. and P. Caldwell (1977), "The Role of Marital Sexual Abstinence in Determining Fertility: A Study of the Yoruba in Nigeria," *Population Studies, 31*, 2, 193–217.

Cantrelle, P. and H. Leridon (1971), "Breastfeeding, Mortality in Childhood and Fertility in a Rural Zone of Senegal," *Population Studies, 25,* 3, 505–533.

Cartwright, A. (1976), *How Many Children?,* Routledge and Kegan Paul, London.

Charbonneaux, H. (1970), "Tourouvre au Perche aux XVII edme et XVIII eme Siecles: Etude de Demographie Historique," *Travaux et Documents, 55,* I.N.E.D., Paris.

Charbonneaux, H. (1979), "Les Regimes de Fecondite Naturelle en Amerique du Nord," in *Patterns and Determinants of Natural Fertility,* H. Leridon and J. Menken, Eds., Ordina Editions, Liege.

Chen, L., S. Ahmed, M. Gesche, and W. H. Mosley (1974), "A Prospective Study of Birth Interval Dynamics in Rural Bangladesh, *Population Studies, 28,* 2, 277–297.

Chowdhury, A. (1978), "Effect of Maternal Nutrition on Fertility in Rural Bangladesh," in *Nutrition and Human Reproduction,* W. Henry Mosley, Ed., Plenum, New York.

Coale, A. J. and T. J. Trussell (1974), "Model fertility schedules: variations in the age structure of childbearing in human populations," *Population Index, 40,* 195–258.

Conception, M. (1981), "Family Formation and Contraception in Selected Developing Countries: Policy Implications of WFS Findings," *World Fertility Survey Conference 1980, Record of Proceedings,* International Statistical Institute, Voorberg, Netherlands.

Delgado, H., A. Lechtig, E. Brineman, R. Martorell, C. Yarbrough, and R. E. Klein (1978), "Nutrition and Birth Intervals Components: The Guatemalan Experience," in *Nutrition and Human Reproduction,* W. Henry Mosley, Ed., Plenum, New York.

Delvoye, J. (1976), "Serum Prolaction in Long-lasting Amenorrhea," *The Lancet, ii,* 288–289.

Erhardt, C. L. (1963), "Pregnancy Losses in New York City, 1960," *American Journal of Public Health, 53,* 9, 1337–1352.

Ford, K. (1978), "Contraceptive Use in the United States 1973–1976," *Family Planning Perspectives, 10,* 5, 264–269.

French, F. E. and J. E. Bierman (1962), "Probabilities of Fetal Mortality," *Public Health Reports, 77,* 10, 835–847.

Frisch, R. E. (1978), "Population, Food Intake and Fertility," *Science, 199,* 22–30.

Gautier, E. and L. Henry (1958), "La Population de Crulai, Paroisse Normande: Etude Historique." *Travaux et Documents, 33,* I.N.E.D., Paris.

Gini, C. (1924), "Premieres recherches sur la Fecondabilite de la Femme," *Proc. Math. Congr.,* Toronto, 889–897.

Van Ginneken, J. K. (1978), "The Impact of Prolonged Breastfeeding on Birth Intervals and on Postpartum Amenorrhea," in *Nutrition and Human Reproduction,* W. Henry Mosley, Ed., Plenum, New York.

Glass, D. V. and E. Grebenik (1954), "The Trend and Pattern of Fertility in Great Britain," *Papers of the Royal Commission on Population, 6,* London, 1954, Part I, p. 255.

Gray, R. (1979a), "Biological Factors other Than Nutrition and Lactation Which May Influence Natural Fertility: A Review," in *Patterns and Determinants of Natural Fertility,* H. Leridon and J. Menken, Ed., Ordina Editions, Liege.

Gray, R. (1979b), "Biological and Social Interactions in the Determination of Late Fertility," Journal of Biosocial Science, Supplement, 6, 97–115.

Gray, R. (1982), "Factors Affecting Natural Fertility Components: Health and Nutrition," in *Determinants of Fertility in Developing Countries: A Summary of Knowledge,* National Academy of Sciences (forthcoming).

Gwatkin, R. (1977), *Fertilization Mechanism in Man and Mammals,* Plenum, New York.

Hartman, C. C. (1962), *Science and the Safe Period,* Williams and Wilkins Baltimore.

Henripin, J. (1954), "La Fecondite de Menages Canadienne an Debut du XVIII-ene Siecle," *Travaux et Documents,* No. 22, INED, Paris.

Henry, L. (1953), "Fondements Theoriques des Mesures de la Fecondite Naturelle," *Review de l'Institut International de Statistique, 21,* 3, 135–252. Translated in *On the Measurement of Human Fertility.* Elsevier, Amsterdam (1972).

Henry L. (1957), "Fecondite et Famille, Models Mathematiques," *Population, 12*, 3, 413–444. Translated in *On the Measurement of Human Fertility*, Elsevier, Amsterdam, 1972.

Henry, L. (1961), "Some Data on Natural Fertility," *Eugenics Quarterly, 8*, 2, 81–91.

Henry, L. (1964), "Mesure du Temps Mort en Fecondite Naturelle," *Population, 19*, 3, 485–514. Translated in *On the Measurement of Human Fertility*, Elsevier, Amsterdam (1972).

Henry, L. (1965), "French Statistical Research in Natural Fertility," in *Public Health and Population Change*, M. C. Sheps and J. C. Ridley, Eds., University of Pittsburgh Press, Pittsburgh.

Henry, L. (1979), "Concepts Actuals et Resultats Empiriques sur la Fecondile Naturelle," in *Patterns and Determinants of Natural Fertility*, H. Leridon and J. Menken, Eds., Ordina Editions, Liege.

Hertig, A. T. (1967), "The Overall Problem in Man," *Comparative Aspects of Reproductive Failure*, K. Benirschke, Ed., Springer-Verlag, New York, p. 11.

Huffman, S. L., A. K. M. Chowdhury, I. Chakraborty, and W. H. Mosley (1978), "Nutrition and Postpartum Amenorrhea in Rural Bangladesh," *Population Studies, 32*, 2, 251–259.

Jain, A. K. (1969a), "Fecundability and Its Relation to Age in a Sample of Taiwanese Women," *Population Studies, 23*, 1, 169–185.

Jain, A. K. (1969b), "Pregnancy Outcome and the Time Required for Next Conception," *Population Studies, 23*, 3, 421–433.

Jain, A. K. (1970), "Demographic Aspects of Lactation and Postpartum Amenorrhea," *Demography, 7*, 2, 255–271.

James, W. H. (1969), "A Note of Correction with Reference to Parameters of the Menstrual Cycle and the Efficiency of Rhythm Methods of Contraception," *Population Studies, 22*, 281–282.

James, W. H. (1979), "The Causes of the Decline in Fecundability with Age," *Social Biology, 26*, 4, 330–334.

Jelliffe, D. B., E. F. P. Jelliffe, F. T. Sai, and P. Senanayaka (1979), *Lactation, Fertility and the Working Woman*, International Planned Parenthood Federation, Winchmore Press, Upshire.

Knodel, J. (1968), "Infant Mortality and Fertility in Three Bavarian Villages: An Analysis of Family Histories from the 19th Century," *Population Studies, 22*, 3, 297–318.

Knodel, J. (1977), "Family Limitation and the Fertility Transition: Evidence from the Age Pattern of Fertility in Europe and Asia," *Population Studies, 31*, 219–249.

Knodel, J. (1978), "Natural Fertility in Pre-industrial Germany," *Population Studies, 32*, 3, 481–510.

Knodel, J. (1979), "Demographic Transition in German Villages," Paper prepared for the Summary Conference on European Fertility, Princeton, July 1979, Mimeo.

Knodel, J. (1982), "Natural Fertility: Age Patterns, Levels, Trends" in *Determinants of Fertility in Developing Countries: A Summary of Knowledge*, National Academy of Sciences (forthcoming).

Konner, M. and C. Worthman (1980), "Nursing Frequency, Gonadal Functions and Birth Spacing Among Kung Hunter-Gathers," *Science, 207*, 788–791.

Leridon, H. (1977), *Human Fertility: The Basic Components*, The University of Chicago Press, Chicago.

Lestaeghe, R. and H. J. Page (1980), "The Postpartum Non-susceptible Period. Development and Application of Model Schedules," *Population Studies, 34*, 1, 143–170.

McFalls, J. (1979), "Frustrated Fertility: A Population Paradox," *Population Bulletin, 34*, 2, Population Reference Bureau.

McKeown, T. and J. Gibson (1954), "A Note on Menstruation and Conception during Lactation," *Journal of Obstetrics and Gynecology* (Britain), *61*, 824–826.

McKinlay, S., M. Jefferys, and B. Thompson (1972), "An Investigation of the Age at Menopause," *Journal of Biosocial Science, 4*, 161–173.

MacMahon, B. and J. Worcester (1966), "Age at Menopause: United States 1960–1961," *U.S. Vital and Health Statistics Monographs*, Series 11, No. 19, U.S. Government Printing Office, Washington.

McNeilly, A. S. (1978), "Effects of Lactation on Fertility," *British Medical Bulletin, 35*, 2, 151–154.

Majumdar, H. and M. Sheps (1970), "Estimators of a Type I Geometric Distribution from Observations on Conception Times," *Demography, 7*, 3, 349–360.

Malkani, P. K. and J. J. Mirchandani (1960), "Menstruation during Lactation," *Journal of Obstetrics and Gynecology/India, 11*, 11–22.

Martinez, G. A. and J. P. Nalezienski (1979), "The Recent Trend in Breastfeeding," *Pediatrics, 64*, 5, 686–692.

Masnick, G. (1979), "The Demographic Impact of Breastfeeding: A Critical Review," *Human Biology, 51*, 2, 109–125.

Metcalf, M. (1979), "Incidence of Ovulatory Cycles in Women Approaching the Menopause," *Journal of Biosocial Science, 11*, 39–48.

Miller, E., J. A. Fortney, and E. Kessel (1976), "Early Vacuum Aspiration: Minimizing Procedures to Nonpregnant Women," *Family Planning Perspectives, 8*, 1, 33–39.

Moghissi, K. S. (1980), "Prediction and detection of ovulation," *Fertility and Sterility, 34*, 2, 89–97.

Nag, M. (1972), "Sex, Culture and Human Fertility: India and the United States," *Current Anthropology, 13*, 2, 231–237.

Nag, M. (1982), "Factors Affecting Natural Fertility Components: Sociocultural Determinants," in *Determinants of Fertility in Developing Countries: A Summary of Knowledge*, National Academy of Sciences (forthcoming).

Nortman, D. (1974), "Parental Age as a Factor in Pregnancy Outcome and Child Development," *Reports on Population/Family Planning, 16*, The Population Council, New York.

Osteria, T. (1976), "Lactation, Amenorrhea and Birth Intervals in an Urban Community in the Philippines," Mimeo.

Page, H. T. and Lesthaeghe, R. (1981), *Childspacing in Tropical Africa: Tradition and Change*, Academic Press, New York.

Pascal, J. (1969), "Quelque Aspects de la Physiologie du Postpartum," Thése pour le Doctorate en Medicine, Nancy France (quoted in H. Leridon, 1977).

Perez, A., P. Vela, R. Potter, and G. S. Masnick (1971), "Timing and Sequence of Resuming Ovulation and Menstruation after Childbirth," *Population Studies 25*, 3, 491–503.

Potter, R. G. (1961), "Length of the Fertile Period," *Milbank Memorial Fund Quarterly, 39*, 1, 132–162.

Potter, R. G. and M. P. Parker (1964), "Predicting the Time Required to Conceive," *Population Studies, 18*, 1, 99–116.

Potter, R. G., J. B. Wyon, M. Parker, and J. E. Gordon (1965). "A Case Study of Birth Interval Dynamics," *Population Studies, 19*, 1, 81–94.

Potter, R. G., J. B. Wyon, M. New, and J. E. Gordon (1965), "Applications of Field Studies to Research on the Physiology of Human Reproduction," *Journal of Chronic Diseases, 18*, 1125–1140.

Retel-Laurentin, A. (1979), "Quelques Elements de la Fecondite Naturelle dans deux Populations Africaines a Faible Fecondite," in *Patterns and Determinants of Natural Fertility*, H. Leridon and J. Menken, Eds., Ordina Editions, Liege.

Romaniuk, A. (1968), "Infertility in Tropical Africa," in *The Population of Tropical Africa*, J. E. Caldwell and C. Okonjo, Eds., The Population Council, New York.

Salber, E., M. Feinleib, and B. MacMahon (1966), "The Duration of Postpartum Amenorrhea," *American Journal of Epidemiology, 82*, 3, 347–358.

Schwartz, D. P. P. M. MacDonald, and V. Heuchel (1980), "Fecundability, Coital Pregnancy and the Viability of Ova," *Population Studies, 34*, 2, 397–400.

REGULATED FERTILITY

Levels and Trends

In the third quarter of this century, fertility declined in each of the world's major continents:[1]

	Total fertility rate			Decline 1955–1975
	1955	1965	1975	
Africa	6.5	6.5	6.4	−0.1
Asia	5.8	5.4	4.6	−1.2
Latin America	5.7	5.5	5.0	−0.9
North America	2.8	2.4	1.8	−1.0
Europe; USSR	2.7	2.5	2.2	−0.5

The largest absolute change took place in Asia where fertility dropped substantially between 1965 and 1975 in the most populous countries, China, India, and Indonesia. Very little change in the childbearing rate occurred in Africa, the least developed and most traditional of the continents.

It is not possible to review here in detail the fertility experience of all of the world's countries. Instead, eight countries have been selected for more intensive discussion in subsequent sections of this chapter. The choice of these populations was largely based on the availability of detailed data on fertility and the proximate determinants from the *World Fertility Survey*. Countries from all continents are included, representing a wide range of levels and trends in fertility. The total fertility rates of the eight countries between 1955 to 1975 are plotted in Figure 3.1. In 1975 the total fertility rate ranged from a high of 8.0 in Kenya (the highest in the world) to a low of 1.8 in the United States. Over the preceding two decades, fertility rose in Kenya, remained virtually unchanged in Pakistan, and declined in the remaining countries. The largest declines took place in Korea and Colombia.

Age Pattern

The age-specific fertility rates of the eight countries are presented in Figure 3.2. The overall pattern is fairly uniform—an inverted U shape with a

[1] Total fertility rates were calculated from data presented in United Nations (1980). First, the total fertility rates for the 5-year periods from 1950–1955 to 1970–1975 were estimated by assuming that the ratios of the general fertility rate to the total fertility rate for these periods are the same as the projected ratio in 1975–1980. The estimates for 1955, 1965, and 1975 were then obtained by interpolation.

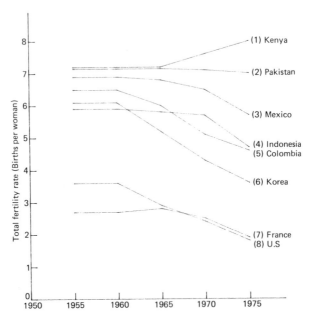

FIGURE 3.1.   Trends in total fertility rates of selected countries. (From United Nations 1980, Bongaarts and Kirmeyer 1982, and Leridon 1981.)

maximum between ages 20 and 30. Kenya and Pakistan have essentially natural fertility because only a few percent of women use contraception or induced abortion. In these two countries the rise in age-specific fertility rates up to age group 25–29 is primarily due to an increase in the proportion of married women, and the decline after age 30 is caused by changes in the proximate determinants of natural marital fertility (sterility, intrauterine mortality, and fecundability). In the six other countries, lower total fertility rates were obtained by lowering the fertility of all age groups. However, the decline is not proportionally the same at all ages. This is evident from Figure 3.2, which plots the age-specific fertility rates as a proportion of the rates observed in Kenya. The largest percentage differences between countries are found at the beginning and end of the reproductive years, resulting in a concentration of childbearing in the central age groups. This compression of the fertility pattern at low levels of overall fertility is caused by a rising age at marriage and by a relatively high prevalence and effectiveness of deliberate fertility control practiced by older women.

Differentials

Table 3.1 presents relative levels of marital fertility by selected background variables. Marital fertility tends to be lowest in the urban, better

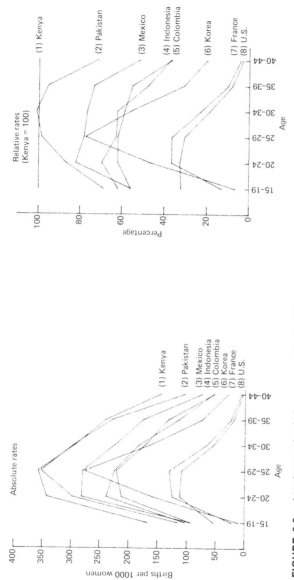

FIGURE 3.2. Absolute and relative age-specific fertility rates. (From Bongaarts and Kirrmeyer 1982, Eurostat 1979, U.S. Bureau of the Census 1978a, 1978c.)

Table 3.1
INDEX OF MARITAL FERTILITY, BY SELECTED BACKGROUND VARIABLES, FOR EIGHT COUNTRIES[a]

	Average	Place of residence		Education of wife				Occupation of husband			
		Rural	Urban	No edu cation	Lower primary	Upper primary	Secon-dary	Agri-culture	Manual work	Sales service	Professional clerk
Kenya (1977)	100	103	83	95	105	100	92	99	101	101	99
Pakistan (1975)	100	99	106	101	97	103	84	99	104	101	97
Mexico (1976)	100	115	85	110	107	82	69	113	103	91	73
Indonesia (1976)	100	98	108	94	106	108	104	92	108	110	106
Colombia (1976)	100	135	79	126	111	77	62	132	85	81	60
Korea (1974)	100	116	88	121	108	98	78	118	94	82	84
France (1977)	100	106	97	--	108	91	91	125	106	95	95
U.S. (1977)	100	111	98	--	127	115	97	133	106	91	93
Average	100	110	93	110	109	97	85	114	101	94	88

a/ Source: For developing countries: Rodriguez and Cleland (1981); for developed countries: United Nations (1976).

educated and higher occupation groups, but there are a substantial number of exceptions to this overall pattern. Contrary to expectations, marital fertility is lower than average in the rural areas of Pakistan and Indonesia, and among women with no education in Kenya and Indonesia. Women whose husband's occupation is in agriculture had below average marital fertility in Kenya, Pakistan, and Indonesia. An explanation for these interesting results will be given in Chapter 5, after differentials in the proximate determinants have been examined.

MARRIAGE

Levels and Trends

Age at first marriage identifies the onset of exposure to the risk of socially sanctioned childbearing, and, as such, it is a principal determinant of the number of births a woman will have. The term *marriage* is used here to refer to all stable sexual unions, including both formal marriages and concensual unions. The mean age at first marriage of females in the mid-1970s averaged 21.4 years for the eight countries in Table 3.2. This average is up from 20.4

Table 3.2
MEAN AGE AT FIRST MARRIAGE FOR FEMALES AND PROPORTION OF FEMALES EVER MARRIED AT AGE 40–44 FOR AVAILABLE DATES IN THE 1960'S AND 1970'S[a]

| | Mean age at first marriage (females) | | Proportion of females ever married at age 40–44 | |
	1960s	mid 1970s	1960s	mid 1970s
Kenya (1969, 1977)	19.1	19.6	97.2	99.0
Pakistan (1961, 1975)	17.5	19.6	97.8	99.0
Mexico (1960, 1976)	21.3	21.7	90.9	94.8
Indonesia (1971, 1976)	19.1	19.8	98.8	99.1
Colombia (1969, 1976)	21.5	22.1	81.5	86.6
Korea (1960, 1974)	21.3	23.1	99.9	99.7
France (1962, 1972)	23.3	22.8	90.6	91.9
U.S. (1960, 1977)	20.5	22.4	93.9	95.3
Average	20.4	21.4	93.8	95.7

[a] Source: The singulate mean ages at marriage were estimated from the age-specific proportions ever married given in: Durch (1980); United Nations (1972, 1976); U.S. Bureau of the Census (1973, 1978a, 1978b, 1978d, 1979a, 1979b, 1979c, 1980).

years in the 1960s, showing a trend toward later marriage. A comparison of countries suggests a tendency for the mean age at marriage to increase with declining fertility (the countries have been ordered according to their level of fertility in Table 3.2). For example, in the mid-1970s, the two countries with highest fertility, Kenya and Pakistan, had a mean age at marriage of 19.6 years, which is about 3 years less than in the two developed countries, France and the United States, where fertility is below the replacement level.

The large majority of women marry at least once during their life in all eight societies. In the mid-1970s, the percentage of women ever married at age 40–44 was very close to 100 in Kenya, Pakistan, Indonesia, and Korea (see Table 3.2.) This percentage is somewhat lower—ranging from 86.6 to 95.3—in the other countries. In Mexico and Colombia, this relatively low proportion ever marrying is probably in part due to underreporting of disruptions of concensual unions which are common in the two societies. That is, some women who experienced a disruption of a concensual union may classify themselves as single rather than as divorced or separated. In the United States and France, a significant proportion of women now decide voluntarily never to marry. Except for an insignificant decline in Korea, the proportion ever married by the end of the reproductive years has risen slightly over time for all countries (see Table 3.2).

Age Patterns

The age-specific proportions currently married among females rise rapidly from near 0 for women under age 15 to a plateau level that is reached in the late twenties or early thirties (see Table 3.3). The large majority of women who ever marry do so between ages 15 and 25. The proportions currently married in the age groups 15–19 and 20–24 are inversely related to the mean age at marriage. Consequently, the lowest proportions married between 15 and 25 are found in France, Korea, and the United States where marriage is relatively late, and the highest proportions are observed in Kenya, Pakistan, and Indonesia. Toward the end of the childbearing years, there appears to be no systematic variation among countries. Most of the eight countries deviate only a few percent from the averages of 85.7% in age group 35–39 and 82.4% in age group 40–44.

The determinants of the age pattern of proportions currently married are the mean age at marriage (mostly in the younger age groups) and the proportion ever marrying and the risks of marital disruption and subsequent remarriage (primarily among older women). Rather than analyzing these determinants separately for each age group, it is simpler to compare the aggregate measures in the last three columns of Table 3.3. These measures separate the reproductive years between ages 15 and 45 into three parts corresponding to the average amount of time spent in the single, married, and previously

Table 3.3

PERCENTAGE OF FEMALES CURRENTLY MARRIED, BY AGE AND AVERAGES OF PERCENTAGES SINGLE, CURRENTLY MARRIED, AND PREVIOUSLY MARRIED[a]

	Age						Average percentage[b] of reproductive years (15-45)		
	15-19	20-24	25-29	30-34	35-39	40-44	Married	Single	Previously married
Kenya (1977)	25.7	73.2	87.3	88.2	86.7	80.6	73.6	16.7	9.7
Pakistan (1975)	38.0	76.0	87.0	92.0	92.0	89.0	79.0	16.3	4.7
Mexico (1976)	17.7	56.7	77.6	83.3	83.4	82.6	66.9	25.9	7.2
Indonesia (1976)	27.5	67.7	83.8	86.7	84.8	77.5	71.3	17.2	11.5
Colombia (1976)	13.7	49.3	69.0	78.6	76.9	74.6	60.3	34.5	5.2
Korea (1977)	3.2	43.7	87.5	94.1	91.5	86.6	67.8	27.4	4.8
France (1977)	4.7	49.3	79.5	85.7	86.4	85.4	65.2	32.0	2.8
U.S. (1977)	9.0	51.3	75.8	82.8	83.5	82.7	64.2	28.1	7.7
Average	17.4	58.4	80.9	86.4	85.7	82.4	68.5	24.7	6.7

a/ Sources: Proportions currently married are taken from Bongaarts and Kirmeyer (1980), Durch (1980), United Nations (1977), and U.S. Bureau of the Census (1978d).

b/ Estimated as average of age specific percentages in each marital state.

Table 3.4
FEMALE MEAN AGE AT FIRST MARRIAGE, BY PLACE OF RESIDENCE AND LEVEL OF EDUCATION (FOR WOMEN MARRIED BEFORE AGE 25 AND AGED OVER 25 AT THE TIME OF THE SURVEY) [a]

| | Place of residence | | Level of education | | |
	Rural	Urban	None	Primary	Secondary
Pakistan	16.9	17.0	16.8	17.7	19.1
Mexico	18.0	19.3	17.2	18.5	20.3
Indonesia	15.6	17.1	15.4	16.0	20.4
Colombia	18.7	19.3	18.0	18.9	19.5
Korea	19.7	20.7	18.0	20.0	21.6
Average	17.8	18.7	17.1	18.2	20.2

[a] From Conception (1981).

married (i.e., widowed, divorced, or separated) state in a synthetic cohort of women.[2] In the eight countries, women are, on average, married for about two-thirds and single for about a quarter of their reproductive years; the remainder is spent in the previously married state. There are, however, significant differences in these measures among the countries. The average proportion single is about 17% in Kenya, Pakistan, and Indonesia, which have the lowest age at marriage and the highest proportions ever marrying (see Table 3.2). In contrast, the overall proportion single is over 25% in the other five countries, where marriage is relatively late and proportions ever marrying relatively low. The average proportion of time in the previously married state is highest in societies where women have been subjected to high risks of widowhood (e.g., in Kenya and Indonesia) or where divorce rates are high (e.g., in the United States). The third measure, the average proportion currently married, can be seen as a residual obtained after removing time in the single and previously married states. It ranges from 60.3% in Colombia to 79.1% in Pakistan and tends to be lowest in the countries with the latest age at marriage.

Differentials

Estimates of the mean age at first marriage, by place of residence and level of wife's education, in five developing countries are given in Table 3.4. On

[2] The synthetic cohorts are assumed to have marital status distributions by age equal to the ones prevailing in the mid-1970s in each country. Estimates of the average time in each marital state are obtained by averaging the corresponding age-specific proportions between ages 15 and 45.

average, urban women marry nearly a year later than their rural counterparts, and women with secondary education are about 3-years older than women without education when they marry for the first time. (The means in Table 3.4 contain a slight downward bias because they are retrospective estimates of women who married before age 25 and are aged between 25 and 49 at the time of the survey, but this bias should not significantly affect the differentials). Urban residence and more education are associated with later marriage in every one of the five countries. The same finding has been reported for all other developing countries for which *World Fertility Survey* data were available in early 1980 (Conception 1981).

CONTRACEPTIVE USE

Levels and Trends

Worldwide, approximately one-third of married women of reproductive age (MWRA) are currently using contraception (Nortman 1980). Contraceptive prevalence varies widely among countries; it is less than 10% in a number of developing countries, and it reaches near 80% in some developed societies. Prevalence trends for selected populations are plotted in Figure 3.3. In all eight countries, contraceptive use increased during the decade from 1965 to 1975, but the rise was so small in Kenya and Pakistan that

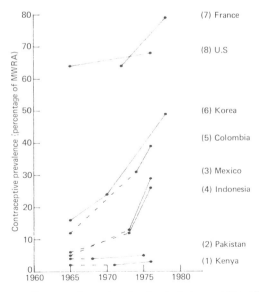

FIGURE 3.3. Contraceptive prevalence trends of selected countries. (From Bongaarts and Kirmeyer 1982; Nortman 1977; Nortman and Holstatter 1980; U.S. Bureau of the Census 1979a, 1979b, 1979c; and Yang and Watson 1974.)

fertility in both countries is still close to natural. Although reliable prevalence statistics are not available for the 1950s, fertility was probably also near natural in the other four developing countries before 1960. This may reasonably be inferred from the fertility trends that indicate that fertility was high and stable in the 1950s (see Figure 3.1) and started to decline in the 1960s when contraceptive prevalence was rising from low levels. The sharpest increments in contraceptive prevalence were observed in Korea, Columbia, Indonesia, and Mexico, the four countries with the most rapid decline in fertility. A comparison of fertility and contraceptive-use levels of the eight countries indicates a high correlation between these two variables (in Figure 3.3, the countries are numbered from highest to lowest total fertility rate [TFR] in 1975). The correlation is not perfect because fertility is also affected by the effectiveness of contraceptive use and by other proximate determinants.

Many different contraceptive methods are available to space births or limit family size. The distribution of contraceptive users by method in Table 3.5 suggests that there is no obvious relationship between overall prevalence and the type of methods used, despite a wide variation in the prevalence of different methods. Apparently, couples in developed countries are generally neither much more nor much less likely to use any given method than couples in developing societies. On average, a little over half of the users take the pill or wear an IUD, about one in eight couples has one partner who has been sterilized, and the remaining one-third uses other methods such as the condom, diaphragm, or spermicides.

Table 3.5
DISTRIBUTION OF CONTRACEPTIVE USERS BY METHOD[a]

	Total	IUD	Pill	Sterilization	Other
Pakistan (1975)	100	12	19	19	50
Mexico (1976)	100	39	52	3	6
Indonesia (1976)	100	21	57	1	21
Colombia (1976)	100	20	32	10	38
Korea (1974)	100	23	25	14	38
France (1978)	100	12	39	6	43
U.S. (1976)	100	9	33	28	30
Average		19	37	12	32

[a] From: Nortman and Hofstatter (1980).

Table 3.6
AGE SPECIFIC PERCENTAGES CURRENTLY USING CONTRACEPTION AMONG MARRIED
WOMEN[a]

	15–19	20–24	25–29	30–34	35–39	40–44
Kenya (1977)	3	6	6	9	6	6
Pakistan (1975)	0	2	5	7	10	7
Mexico (1976)	23	42	46	53	43	34
Indonesia (1976)	13	27	33	34	30	24
Colombia (1976)	26	41	46	56	47	40
Korea (1974)	13	14	28	40	42	34
France (1978)	(60)	72	79	82	83	79
U.S. (1976)	57	70	71	74	70	62
Average	24	34	39	44	41	36

[a] Source: Bongaarts and Kirmeyer (1982), Nortman (1980), Nortman and Hofstatter
(1980). The Korean age-specific fertility rates were estimated with
interpolation from data in World Fertility Survey (1977).

Age Pattern

Age specific prevalence rates for selected countries are given in Table 3.6.
On average, prevalence increases with age until a maximum in age group
30–34 and declines slightly at older ages. As noted in previous studies (e.g.,
Nortman 1980), the age patterns of different populations are similar in shape.
The only significant difference appears to be the relatively high prevalence
among younger women in France and the United States. This presumably
indicates a correspondingly greater inclination to use contraception for spacing purposes.

The leveling off and subsequent decline in prevalence with advancing age
is somewhat surprising, as one would expect a continuous increase in prevalence with age as larger proportions of women reach their desired family
size. One possible explanation for this finding might be that the shape of the
prevalence pattern based on all couples of reproductive age is affected by the
inclusion of pregnant and infecund women who are not exposed to the risk of
contraception. However, if prevalence rates are calculated only for women
exposed to pregnancy risk, the age patterns, although higher, retain their
basic inverted U shape.[3] The cause of the reduction in prevalence at the end

[3] With increasing age, the proportion pregnant declines and the proportions believed to be
infecund increases. These two trends have compensating affects on the pattern of prevalence
among exposed women.

of the reproductive years must be found elsewhere. Perhaps reporting error is a contributing factor. Toward the end of the childbearing years, frequency of intercourse declines and substantial proportions of women have intercourse fewer than once a month. These women may not consider themselves to be current users even if they used contraception the last time they had intercourse. As a result, prevalence rates in the oldest age groups would be biased downward. Yet another explanation may be found in the fact that the age-specific prevalence rates are based on period data that represent different cohorts with different patterns of contraceptive behavior. For example, in each of the six developing countries, women aged 40–44 in 1975 started their childbearing in the 1950s when contraception was virtually absent and deliberate birth control was considered unacceptable. These older cohorts therefore may have been more reluctant to deviate from traditional norms than younger and usually better educated women who initiated their childbearing at a time when the use of contraception was often encouraged by governments.

Differentials

Contraceptive prevalence tends to be higher among urban and educated women than among rural women or those with no education (see Table 3.7).

Table 3.7
PERCENTAGE CONTRACEPTING AMONG MARRIED WOMEN OF REPRODUCTIVE AGE, BY PLACE OF RESIDENCE AND LEVEL OF EDUCATION[a]

| | Place of residence | | Level of education | | |
	Rural	Urban	None	Primary	Secondary
Pakistan(1975)	3	12	4	10	22
Mexico(1976)	11	30	10	20	35
Indonesia(1976)	29	29	24	33	46
Colombia(1976)	27	51	23	41	65
Korea(1974)	31	38	29	34	42
France[b] (1972)	59	65	--59--		68
U.S.[b] (1970)	51	56	--38--		52
Average	30	40	27	34	47

[a] Source: Nortman (1980), United Nations (1976). Estimates for Pakistan and Mexico are based on data presented in Conception (1980), and estimates for Korea are calculated from data in World Fertility Survey (1977).

[b] Excludes sterilization and abstinence.

The average level of current contraceptive use in the seven populations was 30% in the rural compared with 40% in the urban areas, and women without education averaged 27% use, whereas among their counterparts with primary and secondary education prevalence was 34 and 47%, respectively. The consistency of the effect of education and place of residence in these populations is noteworthy. In none of the countries was rural prevalence higher than urban, and better education was without exception associated with more contraceptive use.

CONTRACEPTIVE EFFECTIVENESS

Basic Measures

Before considering available estimates of contraceptive effectiveness, it is necessary to review the definitions of effectiveness and related measures because they are not always used consistently.

Three types of contraceptive effectiveness can be distinguished (Leridon 1977, Tietze and Lewit 1968):

1. *Theoretical effectiveness* (or physiological effectiveness) refers to the effect of a contraceptive under ideal laboratory conditions. It depends solely on the characteristics of the method and is not affected by human error.
2. *Use effectiveness* (also called clinical effectiveness) measures the protection from unintended pregnancy under real-life conditions, allowing for user's carelessness or error as well as method failures.
3. *Extended use-effectiveness* takes into account unintended conceptions following discontinuation of a contraceptive—for example, if it is not well tolerated—in addition to failures during periods of use.

Of these three types of effectiveness, the last two are most widely used. Theoretical effectiveness is difficult to measure, except for the IUD, because it requires perfect compliance from the study population.

The quantitative measurement of contraceptive effectiveness, whether theoretical, use, or extended use, requires the comparison of the pregnancy rates of contraceptors and noncontraceptors in the same population (United Nations 1958). The standard measure of effectiveness (e) equals the proportional reduction in the monthly probability of conception due to use of contraception among fecundable women (Potter 1960, Tietze 1959). Let f_n be the natural fecundability and let f_r be the residual fecundability, then:

$$e = 1 - f_r/f_n \qquad (1)$$

With a perfect contraceptive, the residual fecundability is 0 ($f_r = .0$) and effectiveness is complete: $e = 1.0$. If a totally ineffective method is used, the fecundabilities of contraceptors and noncontraceptors are equal ($f_r = f_n$) and effectiveness is 0: $e = .0$.

Only a few studies provide estimates of effectiveness because of the difficulties encountered in measuring it. However, two related measures of contraceptive failure, the Pearl Index and the cumulative failure rate, are widely available:

—The *Pearl pregnancy rate* (*P*) estimates the number of contraceptive failures per unit of exposure to risk of conception (Pearl 1939).

$$P = \frac{\text{number of undesired pregnancies}}{\text{number of months of exposure to risk}} \times 1200 \qquad (2)$$

The multiplication by 1200 expresses the index as the number of undesired pregnancies per 100 woman years of exposure to risk. This can be interpreted alternatively as the percentage with an undesired pregnancy per year of exposure. For example, a Pearl rate of 10 indicates that 10% of women exposed for an average of a year had a contraceptive failure.

—The *cumulative failure rate* (*F*) equals the proportion of women that becomes unintentionally pregnant within a given time (e.g., a year) from the beginning of a segment of contraceptive use (Potter 1966). The calculation of cumulative failure rates requires the application of fairly complex lifetable methodology (Potter 1966, Tietze and Lewit 1973, Trussell and Menken 1982). In the lifetable, the confounding effects of discontinuation for reasons other than pregnancy are eliminated, so that the (gross) failure rate refers to the experience of a group of women who continuously use contraception except if a pregnancy intervenes.[4] (The 1-year failure rate is analogous to the $_1q_0$ value in the conventional mortality lifetable.)

Of these two measures of contraceptive failure, the latter is often preferred because the Pearl rate has a serious drawback. The problem arises from the fact that the risk of contraceptive failure decreases with duration of use, i.e., women who have been contracepting for say 3 years have a lower risk of failing than women who have used contraception for only a few months (Potter 1960, 1966, Tietze 1959). This phenomenon is caused by differences among women in contraceptive effectiveness and frequency of intercourse (or fecundability). In a group of women initiating contraception, the women with highest frequency of intercourse and lowest effectiveness have the highest risk of conceiving early, thus leaving increasing proportions of women with lower risks over time. As a consequence, the Pearl rate is sensitive to the mixture of durations of exposure that is included in its

---

[4] A distinction can be made between the gross failure rate as defined here and the net failure rate which does not eliminate the confounding effects of discontinuation for reasons other than pregnancy.

measurement. For example, a Pearl rate calculated for 100 years of exposure will be higher if it is based on 1 year of exposure for 100 women, than if it is calculated from data from 20 women with 5 years of exposure each. This problem can be greatly reduced by observing women for a fixed interval of say 1 year, so that all women contribute 12 months of exposure except if they become pregnant or discontinue use. As will be demonstrated, this so-called improved Pearl rate is closely related to the 1-year cumulative failure rate. The term "improved Pearl index" was introduced by Henry (1968).

It should be emphasized that the Pearl rate and the cumulative failure rate are not direct measures of contraceptive (in-)effectiveness. The reason is that the probability of method failure during a given interval of exposure not only depends on the contraceptive effectiveness but also, and equally, on the frequency with which the method is put to the test (i.e., the frequency of intercourse). Clearly, if a method is tested in two groups of women who are identical in every respect except that one has twice the coital rate of the other, then the Pearl index and cumulative failure rate of the former will be twice those of the latter. This problem is not encountered if effectiveness is measured as the proportional reduction in the monthly conception risk (e) because the rate of undesired pregnancy is compared with the rate in the absence of contraception. Residual fecundability f_r, and natural fecundability, f_n, are both functions of the coital rate, but their ratio, which is used to calculate e from Equation (1), is insensitive to the frequency of intercourse.

In summary, a variety of approaches are available to measure the protection from unintended pregnancy provided by contraception. Three different measures—the effectiveness, the Pearl rate, and the cumulative failure rate—can be applied in three different circumstances—theoretical, use, and extended use—yielding a total of nine measures:

1. Theoretical effectiveness
2. Use-effectiveness
3. Extended use-effectiveness
4. Theoretical Pearl pregnancy rate
5. Use–Pearl pregnancy rate
6. Extended use–Pearl pregnancy rate
7. Cumulative theoretical failure rate
8. Cumulative use–failure rate
9. Cumulative extended-use–failure rate

Not surprisingly, clear distinctions between these different measures are not always made in the literature. For example, the (use–) Pearl rate or the cumulative (use–) failure rate are often referred to as measures of use-effectiveness. For reasons just given, this is, strictly speaking, incorrect. At best, the Pearl rate and cumulative failure rates can be called *indirect measures* of (in-)effectiveness, but it would be preferable to use the correct terminology, reserving the term *effectiveness* for measures of the proportional reduction in fecundability.

A dimension of contraceptive performance not captured by effectiveness or failure measures is the continuity of use. The reduction in fertlity obtained in a group of women who initiate contraception depends on the effectiveness of contraception while in use, but also on the duration of use. A widely available indicator of this aspect of contraceptive performance is the continuation rate that measures the proportion of acceptors that still practice contraception at a given duration (say 1 year) after initiating contraception.

Relationships between Measures of Effectiveness and Failure

To allow a comparison of the contraceptive effectiveness and failure rates, it is necessary to base them on the same exposure duration. Using a 1-year exposure interval, a set of equations relating the improved Pearl rate (P') and the 1-year cumulative failure rate (F') to the effectiveness e and natural fecundability f_n is derived in the appendix to this chapter. For example, the following equation for P'

$$P' = 1200 \times f_n \times (1 - e) \tag{3}$$

indicates that the improved Pearl rate varies directly with the natural fecundability and declines with rising levels of effectiveness, as expected. (This equation is valid regardless of whether the theoretical, use, or extended use versions of P' and e are taken.) To illustrate, Table 3.8 provides numerical estimates of P' for a range of values of effectiveness and natural fecundability. The appendix also contains a derivation and empirical validation of the following equation that shows the relationship between the improved Pearl rate and the 1-year cumulative failure rate.

$$F' = 0.01 \times P'/(1 + 0.005 \times P') \tag{4}$$

Based on this equation, corresponding estimates of F' are provided in the last column of Table 3.8.

Estimates of Contraceptive Effectiveness

Because reliable direct estimates of contraceptive effectiveness are extremely difficult to obtain, it is usually necessary to derive effectiveness levels from available estimates of Pearl rates or cumulative failure rates. A detailed study of 1-year cumulative (use–) failure rates has recently been made in the United States from data collected in a 1973 survey of married women of reproductive age (Vaughan, Trussell, Menken and Jones 1977). The cumulative 1-year use–failure rates found in this study ranged from 0.02

Table 3.8
MODEL ESTIMATES OF IMPROVED PEARL PREGNANCY RATES AND CUMULATIVE
1-YEAR FAILURE RATES FOR DIFFERENT LEVELS OF CONTRACEPTIVE EFFECTIVENESS
AND FECUNDABILITY[a]

Contraceptive effectiveness (e')	Estimated improved Pearl pregnancy rate (P')	Estimated cumulative 1-year failure rate (F')
Natural fecundability = 0.05		
1.00	0	0.0
0.95	3	0.030
0.90	6	0.058
0.80	12	0.113
Natural fecundability = 0.15		
1.00	0	0.0
0.95	9	0.086
0.90	18	0.165
0.80	36	0.305
Natural fecundability = 0.25		
1.00	0	0.0
0.95	15	0.140
0.90	30	0.261
0.80	60	0.462

a/ Source: Equations (3) and (4).

for the pill to 0.191 for the users of the rhythm method (see Table 3.9). From these failure rates the corresponding use-effectiveness levels are estimated with an equation derived in the appendix (average natural fecundability is assumed to be 0.14).[5] The results are presented in the last column of Table 3.9.

[5] An age-specific fecundability pattern for the United States is introduced in Chapter 7. This pattern assumes that (natural) fecundability is 0.19 between ages 20 and 30, and declines linearly thereafter from 0.19 at age 30 to 0 at age 48. Averaging this fecundability schedule between ages 22, the approximate age at first marriage in the United States, and age 45 yields an average fecundability of 0.14. This is the value used in the calculation of the effectiveness levels in Table 3.9. It should be emphasized that the resulting use-effectiveness estimates are only approximate because in reality there are likely to be some differences in the fecundability levels of the users of different types of contraception. However, more accurate effectiveness estimates are difficult to make in the absence of measures of method-specific fecundability.

Table 3.9

OBSERVED U.S. CUMULATIVE 1-YEAR USE-FAILURE RATES AND ESTIMATES OF
CORRESPONDING USE-EFFECTIVENESS LEVELS[a]

	Cumulative 1-year use-failure rate	Approximate use-effectiveness
Sterilization	(0.0)	(1.00)
Pills	0.020	0.99
IUDs	0.042	0.97
Condom	0.101	0.94
Diaphragm	0.131	0.92
Foam/Cream/Jelly	0.145	0.91
Rhythm	0.191	0.87
Other	0.108	0.93

[a] Source: Vaughan, Trussell, Menken and Jones (1977) and Equation (12) in
the appendix, assuming $f_n' = 0.14$.

The use effectiveness of the different contraceptives ranges from 1.0 for
sterilization to 0.87 for the rhythm method. Comparable estimates for other
developed countries are not available, but Laing (1978) provides the following method-specific use-effectiveness estimates for the Philippines: pills:
0.95; IUDs: 0.96; rhythm: 0.80; and condom: 0.62.

A comparison of these results with the U.S. figures in Table 3.9 reveals
large differences for pill and condom users, but the effectiveness estimates
for the IUD are nearly the same. One would expect little difference in IUD
effectiveness levels because they are not affected by human behavior (except
for errors in the reporting of IUD expulsions).

There are no reliable data on differentials in contraceptive effectiveness,
but a number of studies of differentials in cumulative failure rates have been
made. In the United States, Vaughan, Trussell, Menken, and Jones (1977)
demonstrate that the failure risk declines with advancing age and that women
who want to prevent another pregnancy have lower failure rates than women
who only want to delay the next pregnancy. After controlling for age and
intention, there no longer appears to be much difference between socioeconomic groups (Vaughan, Trussell, Menken and Jones 1977). Whether these
findings also apply to differentials in use-effectiveness is not clear, because
differences in coital frequency are responsible for some of the variation
in failure rates. It is likely for example, that the decline in failure rate with
age is in part due to the reduction in frequency of intercourse among older
women.

INDUCED ABORTION

Access to legal abortion in different countries depends largely on the extent of restrictions imposed by law. In 1980, the proportions of the world population governed by specific laws were estimated to be as follows (Tietze 1981):

28% Abortion prohibited without exception, or allowed only to save the life of the woman (e.g., majority of countries in Latin America and Africa, and Muslim countries of Asia)

10% Abortion authorized on broader medical grounds to avert threat to woman's health (often including mental health) and on eugenic or juridical (rape, incest) indication (e.g., Korea)

24% Termination of pregnancy allowed on social–medical grounds such as health, unmarried status, or inadequate income (e.g., most of Eastern Europe, Japan, India)

38% Abortion on request, but generally limited to the first trimester of pregnancy (e.g., U.S., USSR, China, France)

The majority of the world's women (62%) live in areas where abortion laws are quite liberal—just over a quarter of the women are governed by restrictive laws. In the remaining 10%, the fairly restrictive laws are not always enforced, as for example in Korea.

Estimates of total abortion rates based on legal abortions reported in all countries with reasonably complete statistics are shown in Table 3.10. (The *total abortion rate* (TA) is defined as the average number of induced abortions per woman at the end of the reproductive years if current age-specific abortion rates prevail throughout the childbearing years). Among the developed countries the total abortion rate is over 1.0 in 5 countries, all in eastern Europe. Intermediate abortion levels with TAs between 1 and .5 are observed in eight countries mostly in eastern and northern Europe. In the remaining 10 developed countries, many in western Europe, the total abortion rate is less than .5. In the developing world the total abortion rate is highest in Cuba and Korea, intermediate in Singapore, and lowest in Tunisia, Hong Kong, and India. China is not included because reliable statistics are lacking. However, abortion is legal and freely available, and, with the governments emphasis on birth control, China's total abortion rate probably exceeds 0.5. Virtually all other, mostly developing, countries not included in Table 3.10 have restrictive laws, and levels of induced abortion are likely to be low or negligible, with the possible exception of some urban areas in Latin America.

Between the early sixties and the late seventies, abortion rates have generally increased. Abortion laws were liberalized in at least 17 countries, which often resulted in substantial increments in the number of abortions. More restrictive laws were adopted in 5 countries, Bulgaria, Czechoslavakia,

Table 3.10

ESTIMATES OF TOTAL ABORTION RATES (TA) IN 1978 OF COUNTRIES WITH REASONABLY RELIABLE ABORTION STATISTICS[a]

Developed countries		
TA above 1.0	TA between 1.0 and 0.5	TA less than 0.5
		Italy 0.47
USSR[b] (5.40)	Czechoslovakia 0.87	Finland 0.47
Rumania 2.57	Japan 0.70	France 0.41
Bulgaria 2.05	U.S. 0.69	England 0.34
Yugoslavia[b] 1.32	East Germany 0.67	Canada 0.34
Hungary 1.11	Denmark 0.67	Iceland 0.26
	Sweden 0.58	Scotland 0.21
	Norway 0.55	West Germany 0.16
	Poland 0.55	Netherlands 0.15
		New Zealand 0.11

Developing countries		
TA above 1.0	TA between 1.0 and 0.5	TA less than 0.5
Cuba 1.56	Singapore 0.87	Tunisia 0.49
Korea[b] 1.50		Hong Kong 0.16
		India 0.06

[a] From: Tietze (1979, 1981). TA estimated as 30 times abortion rate among women aged 15–44.

[b] Estimates for 1969 or 1970.

Hungary, New Zealand, and Romania, causing reductions in abortion rates (Tietze 1979).

Age-specific induced abortion rates typically have an inverted U-shaped pattern. In many Western developed countries, the abortion rate reaches a maximum around age 20, whereas in eastern Europe and in developing countries the highest abortion rates are observed after age 25 (Tietze 1981). These differences are, in part, the consequence of differences in abortion rates between marital status groups. In the West often more than half of all abortions occur among single or previously married women, but in the other countries the majority of abortions take place while women are married.

SUMMARY

A brief overview of levels, trends, age patterns, and socioeconomic differentials in controlled fertility and its proximate determinants is presented in this chapter. Because it was not possible to include data from all countries in the world, a set of eight populations with widely varying levels of fertility and from all of the world's continents is selected for discussion. Among the principal findings are: (a) a general trend toward lower fertility, later marriage, and higher contraceptive prevalence; (b) a close correlation between levels of fertility and contraceptive prevalence; (c) a uniformly negative effect of urban residence and higher education on the level of contraceptive use; and (d) a substantial number of exceptions to the general pattern of lower marital fertility among higher socioeconomic status groups. The section on contraception includes a review of definitions of measures of contraceptive effectiveness and failure. A set of simple equations is derived to relate the contraceptive effectiveness, the cumulative failure rate, and the Pearl pregnancy rate to one another. Problems encountered in the interpretation, use, and measurement of these variables are discussed. Only a few empirical estimates are presented because nationally representative measures of contraceptive effectiveness are not available for most populations.

APPENDIX

The homogeneous case, in which all couples use contraception with equal effectiveness (e) and have the same natural fecundability (f_n), will be considered first. The monthly risk of conception then equals $(1 - e)f_n$. Multiplying this by 1200 yields the risk per 100 years of exposure, the improved Pearl rate, P':

$$P' = 1200 (1 - e)f_n \qquad (1)$$

As noted by Ryder (1973), the probability of not failing in 1 month is $1 - (1 - e)f_n$, and in 12 months it equals $(1 - (1 - e)f_n)^{12}$. The 1-year failure rate, F', therefore equals

$$F' = 1 - (1 - (1 - e)f_n)^{12} \qquad (2)$$

Substitution of (1) in (2) yields

$$F' = 1 - (1 - P'/1200)^{12} \qquad (3)$$

For small values of P' it is easily demonstrated (by expansion into series) that F' estimated by Equation (3) is very closely approximated by

$$F' = 0.01 P'/(1 + 0.005 P') \qquad (4)$$

For example if $P' = 30, F' = .2620$ according to Equation (3) and 0.2609 according to Equation (4). The difference is negligable for all practical purposes. Equation (4) (which is the same as Equation (4) in the text) would be exact if the contraceptive failures are distributed evenly throughout the year. In reality there is a slight concentration of failures in the earlier months, but this apparently produces only a very slight error.

In the heterogeneous case, natural fecundability declines and effectiveness increases over time. Let $P(n), f_n(n)$, and $e(n)$ denote, respectively, the Pearl rate, the natural fecundability and the effectiveness in the nth month after the initiation of a segment of contraceptive use. The improved Pearl rate for the first 12-month period, P', is closely approximated by

$$P' = 1/12 \sum_{n=1}^{12} P(n) \tag{5}$$

In general, Equation (5) gives a slight underestimate of the true value of P' because $P(n)$ is highest in the early months, and the early months contribute slightly more woman years of exposure than the later months. Small values of $P(n)$ and high continuation rates, as well as low rates of decline in $P(n)$ with n, are associated with small errors. That the error caused by applying Equation (5) is typically small can be demonstrated with empirical data from Tietze (1962). He estimates that $P(n)$ values for diaphragm and jelly users declined from 15.4 in the first 3 months, to 12.1 in the second quarter, to 10.0 in the second half of the first year. With Equation (5), the value of P' is estimated at 11.9. This compares with an estimate of 12.1 obtained by Tietze for the Pearl rate in the first year, showing good agreement. (Actually, Tietze's estimate is slightly higher than the true improved Pearl rate because Tietze includes a small number of women whose experience was truncated at less than 1 year by the interview. These should ideally be excluded in the estimation of the improved Pearl rate used here.)

Substituting $P(n) = 1200 (1 - e(n)) f_n(n)$ in Equation (5) produces

$$P' = 1/12 \sum_{n=1}^{12} 1200 (1 - e(n)) f_n(n) \tag{6}$$

With the average effectiveness e' estimated as

$$e' = 1/12 \sum_{n=1}^{12} e(n) \tag{7}$$

and the weighted average fecundability equal to

$$f_n' = 1/12 \sum_{n=1}^{12} (1 - e(n)) f_n(n)/(1 - e') \tag{8}$$

Equation (6) simplifies to

$$P' = 1200 (1 - e') f_n \tag{9}$$

Potter, McCann and Salcoda (1970) have shown that with reasonably effective contraception the values of $f_n(n)$ are virtually constant during the first year. In that case, f_n' equals the unweighted average natural fecundability. The equivalent of Equation (2) in the heterogeneous population is

$$F' = 1 - \prod_{n=1}^{12} (1 - (1 - e(n)) f_n(n)$$

$$= 1 - \prod_{n=1}^{12} (1 - P(n)/1200) \tag{10}$$

For values of $P(n)$ within the normal observed range, an excellent approximation of F' is obtained by substituting the average value P' for $P(n)$ in Equation (10):

$$F' = 1 - \prod_{n=1}^{12} (1 - P'/1200)$$

$$= 1 - (1 - P'/1200)^{12} \tag{11}$$

which is the same as Equation (3). As in the homogeneous case, this can with good approximateion be simplified to Equation (4).

The validity of Equation (4) in the heterogeneous case can be demonstrated empirically with data from Potter (1960). Potter estimates the following Pearl pregnancy rates and cumulative failure rates for the first 12 months of exposure, by stage of family building, from data of the Princeton fertility study:

Family stage	Observed Pearl pregnancy rate	Observed cumulative failure rate	Estimated cumulative failure rate (Equation 4)
Before first pregnancy	38.8	.317 ± .023	.325
Before second and third pregnancy	25.9	.231 ± .016	.229
After second birthspacers	22.2	.208 ± .018	.200
Limiters	5.9	.058 ± .017	.057

Clearly, there are no significant differences between observed and estimated 1-year cumulative failure rates. Similar findings are reported by Trussell and Menken (1982), who estimate the cumulative failure rate from the ordinary 12-month Pearl rate. (The agreement they found between observed and estimated failure rates would have been even better if they had excluded women whose experience was truncated at less than 1 year by the interview.)

Substitution of Equation (9) in (4) yields, after rearranging:

$$e' = 1 - F'/(12f_n' (1 - 0.5F')) \tag{12}$$

This equation is used in Table 3.9, to estimate use-effectiveness levels from 1-year failure rates.

REFERENCES

Bongaarts, J. (1978), "A Framework for Analyzing the Proximate Determinants of Fertility," *Population and Development Review, 4*, 1, 105–132.

Bongaarts, J. and S. Kirmeyer (1982), "Estimating the Impact of Contraceptive Prevalence on Fertility: Aggregate and Age-Specific Versions of a Model," in *The Role of Surveys on the Analysis of Family Planning Programs,* A. Hermalin and B. Entwisle, Eds., Ordina, Liege.

Conception, M. B. (1981), "Family Formation and Contraception in Selected Developing Countries: Policy Implications of WFS Findings," *World Fertility Survey Conference 1980, Record of Proceedings* International Statistical Institute, Voorburg, Netherlands.

Durch, J. S. (1980), "Nuptiality Patterns in Developing Countries: Implications for Fertility," *Reports on the World Fertility Survey, 1,* Population Reference Bureau, Washington.

Eurostat (1979), *Demographic Statistics 1978,* Statistical Office of the European Communities, Brussels.

Henry, L. (1968), "Essay de Calcul de l'Efficacite de la Contraception," *Population, 23,* 2, 265–278.

Laing, J. E. (1978), "Estimating the Effects of Contraceptive Use on Fertility: Techniques and Findings from the 1974 Philippine National Acceptor Survey," *Studies in Family Planning, 9,* 6, 150–162.

Leridon, H. (1977), *Human Fertility: The Basic Components,* The University of Chicago Press, Chicago.

Leridon, H. (1981), "Fertility and Contraception in 12 Developed Countries," *Family Planning Perspectives, 13,* 2, 93–102.

Nortman, D. L. (1977), "Changing Contraceptive Patterns: A Global Perspective," *Population Bulletin, 32,* 3, August, 1–37.

Nortman, D. L. (1980), "Empirical Patterns of Contraceptive Use: A Review of the Nature and Sources of Data and Recent Findings," in *The Role of Surveys in the Analysis of Family Planning Programs,* A. Hermalin and B. Entwisle, Eds., Ordina, Liege.

Nortman, D. L. and E. Hofstatter (1980), "Population and Family Planning Programs," *A Population Council Fact Book,* 10th Ed., The Population Council, New York.

Pearl, R. (1939), *The Natural History of Population,* Oxford University Press, London.

Potter, R. G. (1960), "Length of Observation Period as Affecting the Contraceptive Failure Rate," *The Milbank Memorial Fund Quarterly, 38,* 140–152.

Potter, R. G. (1966), "Application of Life Table Techniques to Measurements of Contraceptive Effectiveness," *Demography, 3,* 2, 297–304.

Potter, R. G., B. McCann and J. Sakoda (1970), "Selective Fecundability and Contraceptive Effectiveness," *Milbank Memorial Quarterly, 48,* 91–102.

Rodriguez, G. and J. Cleland (1981), "Socioeconomic Determinants of Marital Fertility in Twenty Countries; A Multivariate Analysis," *World Fertility Survey Conference, 1980,* Record of Proceedings, International Statistical Institute, Voorburg, Netherlands.

Tietze, C. (1959), "Differential Fecundity and Effectiveness of Contraception," *The Eugenics Review, 50,* 231–237.

Tietze, C. (1962), "The Use-Effectiveness of Contraceptive Methods," in *Research in Family Planning,* C. V. Kiser, Ed., Princeton University Press, Princeton.

Tietze, C. (1979), "Induced Abortion: 1979," *A Population Council Factbook,* The Population Council, New York.

Tietze, C. (1981), Induced Abortion: A World Review 1981, *A Population Council Fact Book*, The Population Council, New York.

Tietze, C. and S. Lewit (1968), "Statistical Evaluation of Contraceptive Methods: Use-Effectiveness and Extended Use-Effectiveness," *Demography*, 5, 2, 931–940.

Tietze, C. and S. Lewit (1973), "Recommended Procedures from the Statistical Evaluation of Intrauterine Contraception," *Studies in Family Planning*, 4, 35–42.

Trussell, J. and J. Menken (1982), "Life Table Analysis of Contraceptive Failure," in *The Role of Surveys on The Analysis of Family Planning Programs*, A. Hermalin and B. Entwisle, Ed., Ordina, Liege.

United Nations (1958), "Multilingual Demographic Dictionary," *Population Studies*, No. 29, Department of Economic and Social Affairs, New York.

United Nations (1972), *Demographic Yearbook 1971*, Department of Economic and Social Affairs, New York.

United Nations (1976), "Fertility and Family Planning in Europe Around 1970," *Population Studies*, No. 58, Department of Economic and Social Affairs, United Nations, New York.

United Nations (1977), *Demographic Yearbook 1976*, Department of Economic and Social Affairs, New York.

United Nations (1980), *Selected Demographic Indicators by Country, 1950–2000*, Department of International Economic and Social Affairs, (ST/ESA/SER.R/38), New York.

U.S. Bureau of the Census (1973), Census of Population, *Detailed Characteristics, United States Summary* PC(1) D1, U.S. Gov't Printing Office, Washington.

U.S. Bureau of the Census (1978a), "Republic of Korea," *Country Demographic Profiles*, ISP-DP-17, June 1978, U.S. Gov't Printing Office, Washington, D.C.

U.S. Bureau of the Census (1978b), "Kenya," *Country Demographic Profiles*, ISP-DP-11, U.S. Gov't Printing Office, Washington, D.C. 1978.

U.S. Bureau of the Census (1978c), *Statistical Abstract of the United States: 1978*, U.S. Gov't Printing Office, Washington, D.C.

U.S. Bureau of the Census (1978d), "Marital Status and Living Arrangements: March 1977" *Annual Population Reports*, Population Characteristics, P-20, no. 328, April 1980; U.S. Gov't Printing Office, Washington D.C.

U.S. Bureau of the Census (1979a), "Indonesia," *Country Demographic Profiles*, ISP-DP-18, May 1979, U.S. Government Printing Office, Washington, D.C.

U.S. Bureau of the Census (1979b), "Mexico," *Country Demographic Profiles*, ISP-DP-14, September 1979, U.S. Gov't Printing Office. Washington, D.C.

U.S. Bureau of the Census (1979c), "Colombia," *Country Demographic Profiles*, ISP-DP-20, October 1979, U.S. Gov't Printing Office, Washington, D.C.

U.S. Bureau of the Census (1980), "Pakistan," *Country Demographic Profiles*, ISP-DP-24, March 1980, U.S. Gov't Printing Office, Washington, D.C.

Vaughan, B., J. Trussell, J. Menken and E. F. Jones (1977), Contraceptive Failure among Married Women in the United States, 1970–1973." *Family Planning Perspectives*, 9 (6), 251–258.

World Fertility Survey (1977), "The Korean National Fertility Survey," *First Country Report*, National Bureau of Statistics of the Economic Planning Board, Seoul, Korea.

Yang, J. and W. B. Watson (1974), "Family Planning and Fertility Decline in Korea, Retrospection and Prospect," in *Population and Family Planning in Korea*, vol. II, Korean Institute for Family Planning, Seoul, Korea.

4

An Aggregate Fertility Model

In Chapter 2 a simple arithmetic model was introduced to analyze the effects of various proximate determinants on natural fertility. Aside from the fact that it relied on a number of simplifying assumptions, this model dealt strictly with natural fertility because modifications allowing for deliberate marital fertility control were difficult to introduce. To remedy this shortcoming, we will now present a different aggregate fertility model that describes the relationship between fertility and the proximate determinants in the general case. The effects of deliberate marital fertility control through contraception and induced abortion will specifically be taken into account. This more comprehensive model focuses on the four principal proximate determinants of fertility: marriage, contraception, induced abortion, and postpartum infecundability. The remaining proximate determinants, natural fecundability, spontaneous intrauterine mortality, and permanent sterility, were earlier shown to be generally much less important causes of variations in fertility, and they will therefore be treated here as secondary factors.

THE STRUCTURE OF THE MODEL

The basic variables and concepts used in the model are summarized in Figure 4.1. The four principal proximate determinants are considered inhib-

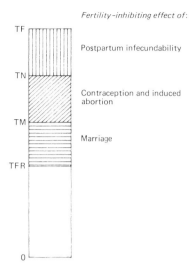

Fertility-inhibiting effect of:

Postpartum infecundability

Contraception and induced abortion

Marriage

FIGURE 4.1. Relationships between the fertility-inhibition effects of proximate variables and various measures of fertility.

itors of fertility because fertility is lower than its maximum value as a result of delayed marriage and marital disruption, the use of contraception and induced abortion, and postpartum infecundability induced by breastfeeding or abstinence. As is illustrated in Figure 4.1, four different types of fertility levels are identified from which the impact of the proximate variables can be derived. With the inhibiting effects of all proximate determinants present, a population's actual level of fertility is observed, measured by the total fertility rate (TFR). (The total fertility rate and the other fertility rates introduced here are expressed in births per woman at the end of the reproductive years and include only legitimate births.) If the fertility-inhibiting effect of delayed marriage and marital disruption is removed without other changes in fertility behavior, fertility will increase to a level TM (the total marital fertility rate). If all practice of contraception and induced abortion is also eliminated, fertility will rise further to a level TN (the total natural marital fertility rate). Removing, in addition, the practice of lactation and postpartum abstinence further increases fertility to what will be called the total fecundity rate (TF). It will be demonstrated later that the fertility rates TFR, TM, and TN vary widely among populations, but that the TFs of most populations fall within the range from 13 to 17 births per woman, with an average near 15. The TF is relatively invariant because the three remaining proximate factors (natural fecundability, spontaneous intrauterine mortality, and permanent sterility) which determine TF usually cause only modest changes in fertility.

The fertility effects of the four most important proximate determinants, proportion married, contraception, induced abortion, and postpartum infecundability, are measured in the model by four indexes: C_m, C_c, C_a, and C_i, respectively. The indexes can only take values between 0 and 1. When there is no fertility-inhibiting effect of a given intermediate fertility variable, the corresponding index equals 1; if the fertility inhibition is complete, the index equals 0:

C_m = index of marriage (equals 1 if all women of reproductive age are married and 0 in the absence of marriage)

C_c = index of contraception (equals 1 in the absence of contraception and 0 if all fecund women use 100% effective contraception).

C_a = index of induced abortion (equals 1 in the absence of induced abortion and 0 if all pregnancies are aborted).

C_i = index of postpartum infecundability (equals 1 in the absence of lactation and postpartum abstinence and 0 if the duration of infecundability is infinite).

Each index (set of indexes) by definition equals the ratio of the fertility levels in the presence and in the absence of the inhibition caused by the corresponding intermediate fertility variable(s) (see Figure 4.1):

$$C_m = \frac{TFR}{TM} \tag{1}$$

$$C_c \times C_a = \frac{TM}{TN} \tag{2}$$

$$C_i = \frac{TN}{TF} \tag{3}$$

This can be rearranged as

$$TFR = C_m \times TM \tag{4}$$

$$TM = C_c \times C_a \times TN \tag{5}$$

$$TN = C_i \times TF \tag{6}$$

to show that the indexes equal the proportions to which fertility is reduced as the result of the corresponding inhibiting effects. It now follows that

$$TFR = C_m \times C_c \times C_a \times C_i \times TF \tag{7}$$

$$TM = C_c \times C_a \times C_i \times TF \tag{8}$$

$$TN = C_i \times TF \tag{9}$$

These equations summarize the basic structure of the model by relating the fertility measures to the proximate determinants.

In the remainder of this chapter, we will first discuss the estimation of the indexes C_m, C_c, C_a, and C_i from measures of the proximate variables. Next, a test of the validity of the model will be made, and the chapter will conclude with a brief analysis of the relationship between the different fertility rates and their proximate determinants.

DIRECT ESTIMATION OF THE FERTILITY EFFECTS OF THE PROXIMATE DETERMINANTS

A major objective of many applications of the model is the estimation of the fertility-inhibiting effects of the proximate determinants as measured by the indexes C_m, C_c, C_a, and C_i. The Equations (1), (2), and (3) could be used for this purpose, but in practice this is often not possible because the required estimates of fertility rates, especially TN and TF, are lacking. In addition, this approach estimates only the product $C_c \times C_a$, so that no separate estimates of C_c and C_a can be made if both contraception and induced abortion are practiced. Fortunately, another approach, described next, is available to estimate the indexes directly from measures of the proximate determinants.

Estimation of C_m from Proportions Currently Married

The index of marriage is determined by the age-specific proportions currently married among females. C_m is not simply equal to the proportion of all women of reproductive age that are married because the fertility impact of marriage also depends on the age distribution of married women. Married women in the central childbearing years contribute more to the TFR than the youngest or oldest women because age-specific marital fertility rates reach their maximum in the central childbearing ages.

To take this age effect into account, the index C_m is estimated as the weighted average of the age-specific proportions of females currently married, with the weights provided by the age-specific marital fertility rates:

$$C_m = \Sigma\, m(a)\, g(a)/\Sigma\, g(a) \tag{10}$$

where

$m(a)$ = age-specific proportions currently married (or in concensual union) among females.

$g(a)$ = age-specific marital fertility rates[1]

---

[1] In illustrations presented in this study, the age-specific marital fertility rate, $g(a)$, is often obtained by dividing the age-specific fertility rate by the proportion of women that is currently married in each age group. This procedure can lead to erratic results for the age group 15–19 because small errors in the proportion married produce large errors in $g(15-19)$, and because

As the numerator of Equation (10) equals TFR and the denominator equals TM, we find that Equation (10) can be written as $C_m = TFR/TM$, which is identical to Equation (1) as expected.

The calculation of C_m with Equation (10) requires estimates of $m(a)$ and $g(a)$. Difficulty in measuring $g(a)$ for age group 15–19 is sometimes encountered because estimates of this variable may be unreliable; see Footnote 1 for a discussion and a simple solution. Measurement problems may also arise in populations with complex cohabitation patterns. For example, in some Caribbean countries a distinction is made between visiting unions, consensual unions, and formal marriages. (In the applications that follow, visiting unions are given one-half of the weight assigned to consensual unions and marriages.) If, as is often the case, estimates of TFR and TM are available, C_m can, of course, be calculated directly with Equation (1). A numerical example of the estimation of C_m for Sri Lanka, 1975, is presented in the first panel of Table 4.1, yielding $C_m = 0.513$.

The index C_m is similar to the index of marriage I_m proposed by Coale (1965). Both indexes show the extent to which marriage is less than universal, but C_m expresses the effect of nonmarriage in terms of a reduction in fertility per women (TFR/TM), whereas I_m measures this effect as a reduction in the crude birth rate.

Estimation of C_c from Contraceptive Prevalence and Use Effectiveness

The index of contraception varies inversely with prevalence and use effectiveness of contraception practiced by couples in the reproductive age groups. If contraceptive practice is absent or completely inefficient, $C_c = 1.0$. With increasing prevalence and effectiveness, C_c declines below 1.0. The following equation for C_c is derived in the Appendix to this chapter:

$$C_c = 1 - 1.08 \times u \times e \tag{11}$$

where

u = proportion currently using contraception among married women of reproductive age (male methods, abstinence other than postpartum, and sterilizing operations are included).

e = average use-effectiveness of contraception.

---

the incidence of premarital conceptions is in many populations not negligible. In addition, the married women in the 15–19 age group are mostly 18- or 19-years-old, and they are, therefore, not representative of the entire age group. To avoid these problems in this book, $g(15–19) = 0.75 \times g(20–24)$ for all populations, when $g(a)$ is used to calculate TM: TM $= \Sigma\, g(a)$. The multiplication factor 0.75 is based on observed marital fertility rates in a set of natural fertility populations presented by Leridon (1977). For the estimation of C_m, this correction of $g(15–19)$ is not made in the numerator of Equation (10) in order to assure the validity of Equation (1). In Sri Lanka (1975), the correction reduces $g(15–19)$ from 552.3 to 293.5.

Table 4.1

SUMMARY OF MEASURES OF THE PROXIMATE DETERMINANTS AND EQUATIONS REQUIRED FOR THE ESTIMATION OF THE INDEXES C_m, C_c, C_a, AND C_i WITH NUMERICAL EXAMPLES FOR SRI LANKA, 1975

Index	Required measures of the proximate determinants	Resulting estimates of indexes
C_m:	$g(a)$ = the age-specific marital fertility rates	
	$m(a)$ = the age-specific proportions of females currently married	

For Sri Lanka, 1975:

	$m(a)$	$g(a)$	
15-19	0.065	(293.5) (552.3) [a]	
20-24	0.380	391.3	
25-29	0.650	295.5	
30-34	0.822	206.8	
35-39	0.856	136.9	
40-44	0.814	44.5	
45-49	0.817	6.9	

$$C_m = \frac{\Sigma\ m(a)\ \times\ g(a)}{\Sigma\ g(a)} = \frac{TFR}{TM}$$

$$= \frac{3.528}{6.877} = 0.513$$

C_c: u = proportion currently using contraception among married women of reproductive age (15-49)

e = average use-effectiveness of contraception

For Sri Lanka, 1975:

$u = 0.32$
$e = 0.84$ [b]

$C_c = 1 - 1.08 \times u \times e$

$= 1 - 1.08 \times 0.32 \times 0.84$

$= 0.710$

C_a: TA = total abortion rate

For Sri Lanka, 1975:

TA = 0.0

$$C_a = \frac{TFR}{TFR + 0.4 \times (1 + u) \times TA}$$

$= 1.0$

C_i: i = mean duration of postpartum infecundability

For Sri Lanka 1975:

i = 14.4 (estimated from duration of lactation with Equation (1), chapter 2)

$$C_i = \frac{20}{18.5 + i} = 0.608$$

[a] See Footnote 1.
[b] See Footnote 2

The coefficient 1.08 in this equation represents an adjustment for the fact that women (couples) do not use contraception if they know or believe that they are sterile. The absence of contraception among such sterile couples implies that the contraception that is practiced is concentrated among the nonsterile couples. The variable u, which measures prevalence among all couples, therefore, has to be inflated by the sterility correction factor to take into account this concentration of contraception. The average correction factor of 1.08 was estimated directly from data on the proportion of women who believed that they were nonsterile in a number of countries (Nortman 1980).

Estimates of u needed for the calculation of C_c are available from recent fertility or contraceptive prevalence surveys in a large number of populations. In contrast, estimates of the average use-effectiveness, e, are virtually nonexistent. As was noted in Chapter 3, reasonably reliable method-specific use-effectiveness data are only available in two countries, the United States and the Philippines. Until additional data become available, use-effectiveness levels in other populations can only be approximated by relying on the data from these two countries. In the applications that follow, slightly adjusted method-specific use-effectiveness values of the Philippines will be assumed to prevail in developing countries, whereas in the developed countries the levels of the United States will be used.[2] Although this procedure for estimating e is clearly only approximate, the results appear to be acceptable in many applications because use-effectiveness levels of different methods probably vary much less over time and among populations than levels of prevalence u. An illustration of the calculation of C_c for Sri Lanka, 1975, is given in the second panel of Table 4.1.

---

[2] Average use-effectiveness, e, is estimated as the weighted average of the method specific use-effectiveness levels, $e(m)$, with the weights equal to the proportion of women using a given method, $u(m)$: $e = \Sigma\, e(m)\, u(m)/u$. For Sri Lanka, 1975:

	$u(m)$	$e(m)$
Pill	0.019	0.90
IUD	0.048	0.95
Sterilization	0.099	1.00
Other	0.154	(0.70)
	0.32	

so that $e = (0.019 \times 0.9 + 0.048 \times 0.95 + 0.099 \times 1.0 + 0.154 \times 0.7)/0.32 = 0.842$. The $e(m)$ values in this calculation are adapted from a study by Laing (1978) in the Philippines. Laing gives the following effectiveness estimates: 0.949 for the pill; 0.963 for the IUD; 0.798 for rhythm; and 0.616 for the condom. Preliminary evidence from as yet unpublished studies in other developing countries indicates that the use-effectiveness of the pill is lower than in the Philippines. A possible explanation for this finding is that literary levels in the Philippines are among the highest in the developing world. The average effectiveness levels in the developing world used here are therefore estimated to be slightly lower than in the Philippines.

Estimation of the Index C_a from the Total Abortion Rate

To obtain an estimate of the reduction in fertility caused by a given rate of induced abortions, we have to rely here on existing research findings. Typically, the calculation of the number of births averted per induced abortion involves the application of complex mathematical models. The most detailed studies of this topic have been made by Potter (1972), who has demonstrated that:

On average, an induced abortion averts less than one birth. There are two principal explanations for this finding. First, an induced abortion may be unnecessary because a spontaneous abortion or still birth would have prevented the pregnancy from ending in a live birth. Second, and more importantly, with an induced abortion, a woman resumes ovulation much sooner than would have been the case if she had carried the pregnancy to term, especially if the pregnancy would have been followed by a prolonged period of infecundability. The net fertility effect of an induced abortion has to take into account the probability of another conception during the period in which the woman would have been unable to conceive if she had had no induced abortion.

The number of births averted per induced abortion is largely independent of the age of the woman.

The number of births averted per induced abortion is strongly related to the practice of contraception following the induced abortion. In the absence of contraception, an induced abortion averts about 0.4 births, while about 0.8 births are averted when moderately effective contraception is practiced.

To generalize from this last finding, the average number of births averted per induced abortion, b, may be approximated with the equation:

$$b = 0.4 (1 + u) \tag{12}$$

yielding $b = 0.4$ when $u = 0$ and $b = 0.8$ when $u = 1.0$[3]

A convenient overall measure of the incidence of induced abortion is the total abortion rate (TA), equal to the average number of induced abortions per woman at the end of the reproductive period if induced abortion rates remain at prevailing levels throughout the reproductive period (excluding induced abortions to women who are not married). The reduction in fertility

---

[3] In the applications that follow u is taken to equal the prevalence of contraception among all married women. Equation (12) gives usually a good approximation because there is a strong correlation between u and i. If i is known, a more accurate estimate of b would be the ratio of the reproductive time lost per abortion to the birth interval in the absence of contraception. Assuming abortion takes place at 3 months from IMP and using the same birth interval components as in Equation (14), yields $b = 14/(18.5 + i)$. This gives results close to those obtained with Equation 12 for the populations in Table 4.2.

associated with a given level of the TA is calculated as $b \times$ TA, the average number of births averted per woman by the end of the reproductive years. The observed TFR in a population is $b \times$ TA births less than would be the case without induced abortion. The index of induced abortion is now defined as the ratio of the observed TFR to the estimated TFR without induced abortion (TFR $+ b \times$ TA):

$$C_a = \frac{TFR}{TFR + b \times TA} = \frac{TFR}{TFR + .4 \times (1 + u) \times TA} \tag{13}$$

In general, the calculation of index C_a requires estimates of the TFR and the prevalence of contraceptive use u, in addition to the TA. Of course, $C_a = 1.0$ if the TA is 0.

Estimation of the Index C_i from the Duration of Postpartum Infecundability

The index C_i equals the ratio of the TNs in the presence and absence of postpartum infecundability caused by breastfeeding or abstinence. To estimate this ratio, we will make use of the simple reproductive model, introduced in Chapter 2. This model estimates the TN as the number of birth intervals that can be fitted between age 15 and the end of the childbearing years. As postpartum infecundability does not influence the duration of the reproductive years, its effect on fertility operates entirely through modification of the birth interval. The ratio of natural fertility in the presence and absence of postpartum infecundability, therefore, equals the ratio of the average birth interval without and with postpartum infecundability. If no breastfeeding and postpartum abstinence are practiced, the birth interval averages about 20 months, the sum of 1.5 months of minimum postpartum anovulation, 7.5 months of waiting time to conception, 2 months of time added by spontaneous intrauterine mortality, and 9 months for a full-term pregnancy (see Chapter 2). In the presence of breastfeeding and postpartum abstinence, the average birth interval equals, approximately, 18.5 months (7.5 + 2 + 9) plus the duration of postpartum infecundability. The index C_i is now estimated as

$$C_i = \frac{20}{18.5 + i} \tag{14}$$

where

i = average duration of postpartum infecundability caused by breastfeeding or postpartum abstinence.

Unfortunately, estimates of i are not as readily available as measures of the other principal proximate determinants. But in populations where estimates of the average duration of breastfeeding exist, an approximate duration of postpartum amenorrhea can be estimated with Equation (1) in Chapter 2. The last panel of Table 4.1 presents the calculation of C_i for Sri Lanka, 1975.

The Effects of the Remaining Proximate Determinants

The fertility-inhibiting impact of the four principal proximate determinants are explicitly taken into account in the model through the indexes C_m, C_c, C_a, and C_i, which have just been described. The remaining proximate determinants, the waiting time to conception, the risk of intrauterine mortality, and the onset of permanent sterility, are not separately represented in the model by indexes. Instead, the combined effect of these three factors is measured by the TF. The distinction between the four principal and the three secondary proximate determinants is made on the basis of the analysis in Chapter 2, which showed that variations in the secondary factors generally have relatively little influence on fertility. As a consequence, the TF can be expected to vary only modestly among populations or over time in the same population, except in unusual cases.

A rough estimate of the average value of the TF can be obtained with the following simple calculation. In the absence of contraception, induced abortion, breastfeeding, and postpartum abstinence, the average birth interval equals about 20 months (see previous section). In the 25 years of childbearing that are available between age 15 and the average at the end of the childbearing years at age 40, a woman would bear 15 children if the average birth interval is 20 months. This estimate of TF = 15 is an approximation, and in Chapter 5 a more accurate estimate of TF = 15.3 will be made on the basis of a detailed empirical analysis. As already noted, differences among populations in natural fecundability, spontaneous intrauterine mortality, or permanent sterility can cause differences in the TF, but the large majority of populations can be expected to have TFs between 13 and 17 births per woman (Bongaarts 1978). Lower TFs are only found in exceptional cases, such as in populations with a high incidence of disease-induced sterility or in populations where spousal separation is unusually frequent or prolonged.

TESTING THE VALIDITY OF THE MODEL

In the preceding section, a set of equations was proposed to estimate the indexes C_m, C_c, C_a, and C_i from the corresponding proximate determinants. Variations in fertility were considered to be largely due to variations in only four factors: the proportions married, contraceptive prevalence and effectiveness, the incidence of induced abortion, and the duration of postpartum infecundability. The remaining, generally much less important, proximate determinants of fertility were represented in the model by the TF, which has values around 15.3 births per woman. The validity of these findings will now be tested by comparing the observed TFRs of different populations with the model estimates of TFRs obtained from the following equation (from Equation [7], assuming TF = 15.3):

$$TFR = C_m \times C_c \times C_a \times C_i \times 15.3 \qquad (15)$$

The testing procedure will be applied in 41 developing, developed, and historical populations, and involves four successive steps: (a) the estimation of the proximate determinants; (b) the calculation of the indexes; (c) the estimation of the TFRs using Equation (15); and (d) a comparison of the model

Table 4.2
ESTIMATES OF THE TFR, TM, AND PROXIMATE DETERMINANTS FOR SELECTED POPULATIONS[a,b]

	Total fertility rate (TFR)	Total marital fertility rate (TM)	Prevalence of contraceptive use (u)	Use effectiveness (e)	Total induced abortion rate (TA)	Months of postpartum infecundability (i)
Developing countries						
Bangladesh, 1975	6.34	7.43	0.08	0.82	---	18.61
Colombia, 1976	4.57	7.91	0.39	0.84	---	5.28
Costa Rica, 1976	3.69	6.46	0.64	0.86	---	3.60
Dominican Rep. 1975	5.85	9.74	0.32	0.89	---	4.76
Guatemala, 1972	7.05	9.74	0.03	0.87	---	14.18
Hong Kong, 1978	2.26	4.56	0.72	0.86	---	3.01
Indonesia, 1976	4.69	6.64	0.26	0.87	---	16.16
Jamaica, 1976	4.32	7.99	0.40	0.84	---	4.25
Jordan, 1976	7.41	9.95	0.24	0.84	---	6.50
Kenya, 1976	8.02	10.44	0.03	0.75	---	11.22
Korea, 1970	3.97	6.85	0.24	0.89	1.5	11.90
Lebanon, 1976	4.77	8.28	0.35	0.83	---	7.14
Malaysia, 1974	4.76	7.84	0.33	0.85	---	3.80
Mexico, 1976	5.73	9.40	0.29	0.86	---	5.28
Nepal, 1976	6.37	7.48	0.02	0.94	---	17.86
Pakistan, 1975	7.02	8.94	0.05	0.83	---	12.65
Panama, 1976	4.57	7.14	0.54	0.90	---	4.25
Peru, 1977	5.11	8.92	0.31	0.78	---	7.85
Philippines, 1976	5.01	8.17	0.35	0.78	---	7.85
Sri Lanka, 1975	3.53	6.88	0.32	0.84	---	14.39
Syria, 1973	7.00	9.59	0.22	0.87	---	8.90
Thailand, 1975	4.70	7.48	0.33	0.91	---	11.80
Turkey, 1968	5.60	7.37	0.35	0.80	---	8.90
Developed countries						
Denmark, 1970	1.78	3.21	(0.70)	0.96	0.169	(3.0)
Finland, 1971	1.61	3.13	(0.80)	0.96	0.284	(3.0)
France, 1972	2.21	4.26	(0.67)	0.94	0.093	(3.0)
Hungary, 1966	1.80	2.92	(0.67)	0.93	2.086	(3.0)
Poland, 1972	2.09	4.78	(0.60)	0.91	0.427	(3.0)
U.K., 1967	2.38	3.91	(0.72)	0.95	0.039	(3.0)
U.S., 1967	2.34	3.71	0.72	0.96	0.004	(3.0)
Yugoslavia, 1970	2.11	3.69	(0.62)	0.95	1.080	(3.0)

Continued

Table 4.2 (continued)

	Total fertility rate (TFR)	Total marital fertility rate (TM)	Prevalence of contra-ceptive use (u)	Use effec-tiveness (e)	Total induced abortion rate (TA)	Months of postpartum infecundability (i)
Historical populations						
Bavarian Villages 1700-1850	(4.45)	11.89	---	---	---	4.9
Crulai 1674-1742 c/	5.60	9.89	---	---	---	11.2
Grafenhausen 1700-1850	(4.74)	10.73	---	---	---	11.3
Hutterites	9.50	12.96	---	---	---	6.0
Ile de France 1740-1779	6.10	12.08	---	---	---	9.6
Oschelbron 1700-1850	(5.06)	10.60	---	---	---	9.0
Quebec 1700-1730 c/	8.00	12.72	---	---	---	6.2
Tourouvre 1665-1714 c/	6.00	10.15	---	---	---	8.2
Waldeck Villages 1700-1850	(4.41)	9.97	---	---	---	11.1
Werdum 1700-1850	(3.78)	9.37	---	---	---	12.7

a/ See Footnote 4.
b/ Figures in brackets are approximate.
c/ Marriages.

estimates of TFR with the observed TFRs to determine how well the four principal proximate determinants predict the fertility level of a population.

Table 4.2 presents the estimates of the proximate determinants (rather than including the entire $m[a]$ distribution, the values for TFR and TM are given, from which C_m is calculated with Equation [1]). The data are obtained from a variety of sources including the *World Fertility Survey*.[4] Estimates of the duration of postpartum infecundability were the most difficult to

[4] Estimates for developed countries and historical populations were taken from Bongaarts (1982) except the contraceptive prevalence data which were inflated to include sterilizing operations for noncontraceptive reasons [in European countries, 3% was added for lack of direct estimates of the incidence of such operations] and the contraceptive effectiveness estimates that were revised in accordance with the method-specific estimates given in Chapter 3. Estimates for developing countries are from Bongaarts and Kirmeyer (1982) except Korea (which is based on Bongaarts [1978] with fertility estimates updated from Cho [1973]).

obtain, and indirect estimation procedures had to be applied in nearly all the populations. For *World Fertility Survey* countries, information about the average duration of breastfeeding was available from which the infecundable interval was obtained with Equation (1) in Chapter 2. For the historical populations, the infecundable interval was derived from the average difference between the marriage to first birth interval and subsequent birth intervals.

From the data in Table 4.2, one can calculate the indexes C_m, C_c, C_a, and C_i with Equations (1), (11), (13), and (14). The results are presented in Table 4.3. The TFRs can now be estimated from the indexes using Equation (15). These model estimates of TFR are given in the last column of Table 4.3.

Table 4.3
ESTIMATES OF THE INDEXES OF THE PROXIMATE DETERMINANTS AND THE MODEL ESTIMATE OF THE TOTAL FERTILITY RATES FOR SELECTED POPULATIONS[a]

	Index of marriage (C_m)	Index of contraception (C_c)	Index of abortion (C_a)	Index of postpartum infecundability (C_i)	Model estimate of total fertility rate (TFR)
Developing countries					
Bangladesh, 1975	0.853	0.929	(1.0)	0.539	6.54
Colombia, 1976	0.578	0.646	(1.0)	0.841	4.80
Costa Rica, 1976	0.571	0.406	(1.0)	0.905	3.21
Dominican Rep. 1975	0.601	0.692	(1.0)	0.860	5.47
Guatemala, 1972	0.724	0.972	(1.0)	0.612	6.59
Hong Kong, 1978	0.496	0.331	(1.0)	0.930	2.34
Indonesia, 1976	0.706	0.756	(1.0)	0.577	4.71
Jamaica, 1976	0.541	0.637	(1.0)	0.879	4.63
Jordan, 1976	0.745	0.782	(1.0)	0.800	7.13
Kenya, 1976	0.768	0.976	(1.0)	0.673	7.72
Korea, 1970	0.580	0.769	0.82	0.658	3.81
Lebanon, 1976	0.576	0.686	(1.0)	0.780	4.72
Malaysia, 1974	0.607	0.697	(1.0)	0.897	5.81
Mexico, 1976	0.610	0.731	(1.0)	0.841	5.73
Nepal, 1976	0.852	0.980	(1.0)	0.550	7.02
Pakistan, 1975	0.785	0.955	(1.0)	0.642	7.37
Panama, 1976	0.640	0.475	(1.0)	0.879	4.09
Peru, 1977	0.573	0.739	(1.0)	0.759	4.92
Philippines, 1976	0.613	0.705	(1.0)	0.759	5.02
Sri Lanka, 1975	0.513	0.710	(1.0)	0.608	3.39
Syria, 1973	0.730	0.793	(1.0)	0.730	6.47
Thailand, 1975	0.628	0.676	(1.0)	0.660	4.29
Turkey, 1968	0.760	0.698	(1.0)	0.730	5.92
Developed countries					
Denmark, 1970	0.555	(0.274)	0.939	(0.930)	2.03
Finland, 1971	0.514	(0.171)	0.887	(0.930)	1.11
France, 1972	0.519	(0.320)	0.973	(0.930)	2.30
Hungary, 1966	0.617	(0.327)	0.564	(0.930)	1.62
Poland, 1972	0.437	(0.410)	0.884	(0.930)	2.26
U.K., 1967	0.609	(0.261)	0.989	(0.930)	2.24
U.S., 1967	0.631	0.254	0.999	(0.930)	2.27
Yugoslavia, 1970	0.572	(0.364)	0.751	(0.930)	2.22

Continued

Table 4.3 (continued)

	Index of marriage (C_m)	Index of contraception (C_c)	Index of abortion (C_a)	Index of postpartum infecundability (C_i)	Model estimate of total fertility rate (TFR)
Historical populations					
Bavarian villages 1700–1850	(0.374)	(1.0)	(1.0)	0.856	4.89
Crulai 1674–1742 b/	0.566	(1.0)	(1.0)	0.673	5.83
Grafenhausen 1700–1850	(0.442)	(1.0)	(1.0)	0.671	4.54
Hutterites 1921–1930 b/	0.733	(1.0)	(1.0)	0.816	9.15
Ille de France 1740–1778 b/	0.505	(1.0)	(1.0)	0.712	5.50
Oschelbron 1700–1850	(0.477)	(1.0)	(1.0)	0.727	5.31
Quebec 1700–1730	0.629	(1.0)	(1.0)	0.810	7.80
Tourouvre 1664–1714	0.591	(1.0)	(1.0)	0.749	6.77
Waldeck Villages 1700–1850	(0.442)	(1.0)	(1.0)	0.676	4.57
Werdum 1700–1850	0.403	(1.0)	(1.0)	0.640	3.95

a/ Figures in brackets are approximate.
b/ Marriages.

A comparison of the model estimates with the observed TFRs reveals that there is good agreement between these two fertility levels (see Figure 4.2). In fact, the model estimates of TFR, and therefore the four principal proximate determinants, explain 96% of the variation in the observed fertility rate. The standard error of the model estimate is 0.36, and in only two populations (Tourouvre au Perche and Malaysia) are the differences more than twice this standard error. Clearly, the earlier conclusion that proportions married, contraception, induced abortion, and postpartum infecundability are the most important proximate determinants of fertility is supported by this finding. These results also confirm the general validity of the model.

The variance in fertility that is not explained by the four principal proximate determinants is due to several factors, including:

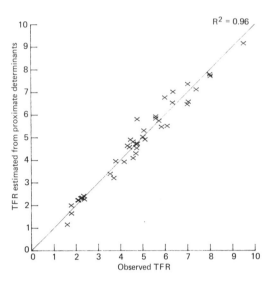

FIGURE 4.2.   Observed and model estimates of total fertility rates of 41 populations.

1. Errors in the measurement of the proximate determinants given in Table 4.2

2. Errors in the specification of the model. To arrive at a simple analytic model for the relationship between fertility and the proximate determinants, a number of simplifying assumptions had to be made. These assumptions made the model less than fully accurate.

3. Deviations from the TF of 15.3. The TF is a function of the three proximate determinants not explicitly included in the model (i.e., natural fecundability, intrauterine mortality, and the prevalence of permanent sterility). As a consequence, the assumption that TF = 15.3 is only an approximation. As already noted, the normal range of TF is from 13 to 17 births per woman.

4. Errors in the observed TFRs. As existing methods for measuring fertility are not perfect, it follows that the best available fertility estimates differ somewhat from the true rates.

5. Induced abortion is assumed absent except in the developed countries and in Korea (a low level of induced abortion common to all populations is allowed for in the estimate of TF = 15.3). If incorrect, this assumption results in an upward bias in the model estimates of TFR.

6. All births are assumed to be legitimate except in the developed countries, where the TFRs given in Table 4.2 are corrected to exclude illegitimate births. In the developing countries in which this assumption is incorrect, the observed TFRs are overestimated.

Although the overall fit of the model is quite good, the combined effect of these error components is sufficiently large to make Equation (15) unsuitable for the accurate estimation of fertility levels. Errors exceeding .5 births per woman in the TFR are not unusual, and other existing methods for estimating fertility are therefore preferable. The purpose of this equation is not to provide a new estimation method; instead, it gives an approximate breakdown of the contributions made by different proximate determinants to levels and trends in fertility.

THE PROXIMATE DETERMINANTS OF FERTILITY LEVELS TF, TN, TM, AND TFR

Having demonstrated that a fair degree of confidence in the model is warranted, we can proceed with an analysis of the general relationship between fertility and the proximate determinants. For this purpose a set of equations for estimating the fertility rates TF, TN, TM, and TFR will be used. It is assumed that only measures of the indexes C_m, C_c, C_a, and C_i are available for the estimation of these fertility levels (it will be shown at the end of this section that more accurate estimates of fertility can be made if at least one of the fertility levels is known in addition to the measures of the indexes). In that case, the following equations are obtained by substituting TF = 15.3 in Equations (7), (8), and (9):

$$TF = 15.3 \tag{16}$$

$$TN = 15.3 \times C_i \tag{17}$$

$$TM = 15.3 \times C_c \times C_a \times C_i \tag{18}$$

$$TFR = 15.3 \times C_m \times C_c \times C_a \times C_i \tag{19}$$

Needless to say, these equations provide only approximate values for TF, TN, TM, and TFR, primarily because they assume that the TF is fixed at 15.3. Nevertheless, these equations provide a very simple and for many purposes adequate tool for analyzing the effects of the proximate determinants on fertility rates, TN, TM, and TFR. We will now briefly discuss the principal causes of variations in each of these fertility levels.

TN

Substitution of Equation (14) in Equation (17) yields:

$$TN = 15.3 \times 20/(18.5 + i) \tag{20}$$

According to this equation, the TN is inversely related to the average duration of postpartum infecundability. Substitution of different values of i produces the estimates of TN given in the last column of Table 4.4. Clearly, postpartum infecundability has a powerful fertility-inhibiting effect. As i in-

Table 4.4

MODEL ESTIMATES OF THE TOTAL NATURAL MARITAL FERTILITY RATE FOR DIFFERENT DURATIONS OF POSTPARTUM INFECUNDABILITY[a]

Duration of postpartum infecundability	Index C_i	Total natural marital fertility rate (TN) [b]
1.5	1.00	15.3 (13.0 - 17.0)
3.0	.930	14.2 (12.1 - 15.8)
6.0	.816	12.5 (10.6 - 13.9)
9.0	.727	11.1 (9.5 - 12.4)
12.0	.656	10.0 (8.5 - 11.1)
15.0	.597	9.1 (7.8 - 10.1)
18.0	.548	8.4 (7.1 - 9.3)
21.0	.506	7.7 (6.6 - 8.6)
24.0	.471	7.2 (6.1 - 8.0)

[a] Source: Equation (20).
[b] Range of TN is obtained by assuming TF to vary from 13 to 17.

creases from its biological minimum of 1.5 months to 2 years, the total TN is more than cut in half, from 15.3 to 7.2 births per woman.

TM

Equation (18) can be analyzed in a similar fashion by substituting Equations (11), (13), and (14) in it. Assuming for simplicity that we are dealing with a country in which no induced abortion is practiced $(C_a = 1.0)$ we obtain:

$$TM = 15.3 \times (1 - 1.08 \times e \times u) \times 20/(18.5 + i) \qquad (21)$$

Based on this equation, Table 4.5 presents estimates of TM for a wide range of values of u and i and for one value, $e = 0.85$, of the usually rather stable use-effectiveness of contraception ($e = 0.85$ is a typical value for the developing countries, see Table 4.2). As expected, the TM has a wide range and is inversely related to the prevalence of contraceptive use and to the duration of postpartum infecundability. An increase in prevalence from 0 to 0.8 reduces marital fertility by three-fourths for all durations of infecundability, and a shortening of the infecundable interval from 24 to 3 months doubles marital fertility independent of the level of contraceptive use. The results in Table 4.5 also show that a given level of marital fertility can be obtained by different combinations of prevalence and duration of infecundability. For example, a population will have a TM of 6.4 if $u = 0.6$ and $i = 3.0$ months, but also if $u = 0.4$ and $i = 12$ months (again assuming $C_a = 1.0$ and $e = 0.85$). Consequently, populations with the same level of marital fertility will not necessarily, and in fact only rarely, have the same proximate determinants.

Over the course of the demographic transition, a population's marital fertility declines. This decline is usually accompanied by large increases in prevalence of contraception from previously low levels and by a shortening of the duration of postpartum infecundability from the intermediate or long intervals found in the pre-transition period. This transition corresponds to a move from the upper right-hand corner to a point in the lower left-hand corner of Figure 4.3 which plots the data in Table 4.5. As an example, the transition from Point A (TM $= 8.4$, $u = 0$, and $i = 18$) to Point B will be considered, with emphasis on the processes in the early phase of the transition. In Figure 4.3, four types of possible transition paths from A to B are plotted.

Path a: The first part of this path follows the line $u = 0$ because only the duration of postpartum infecundability is assumed to change. The result is a temporary increase in marital fertility. Later in the transition, marital fertility declines as contraceptive use increases. Kenya may be an example of a country with approximately this pattern of fertility change.

Path b: The initial phase of this transition is characterized by a decline in the postpartum infecundability accompanied by a compensatory rise in contraceptive use, resulting in a constant marital fertility level during this phase.

Path c: The prevalence of contraception, the duration of postpartum infecundability, the level of marital fertility all change gradually throughout this transition.

Table 4.5
MODEL ESTIMATES OF THE TOTAL MARITAL FERTILITY RATE FOR DIFFERENT DURATIONS OF POSTPARTUM INFECUNDABILITY AND LEVELS OF PREVALENCE OF CONTRACEPTIVE USE[a]

Prevalence of contraceptive use (u)	Duration of postpartum infecundability (months)				
	3.0	6.0	12.0	18.0	24.0
0.0	14.22	12.48	10.04	8.38	7.21
0.2	11.61	10.19	8.20	6.84	5.89
0.4	9.00	7.90	6.35	5.30	4.56
0.6	6.39	5.61	4.51	3.76	3.24
0.8	3.77	3.31	2.67	2.23	1.91

[a] Source: Equation (21).

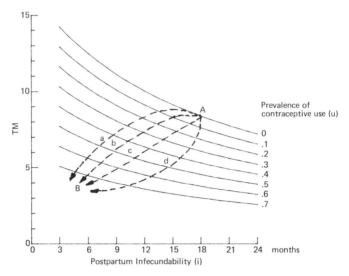

FIGURE 4.3. Total marital fertility rate as a function of the duration of postpartum infecundability and the prevalence of contraceptive use. See text for further explanation.

Path d: In this example, no change takes place initially in the duration of postpartum infecundability, so the entire early decline in marital fertility is attributable to the increase in contraceptive use. The change in fertility in SriLanka may have followed this pattern closely.

It is clear from these examples that not all demographic transitions necessarily have the same continuous decline in marital fertility. A temporary increase in marital fertility is possible if contraceptive use does not increase rapidly enough to offset the positive fertility effect of a decline in the practices of lactation or postpartum abstinence. Such an increase has indeed been observed during part of the transition in a few populations (Knodel 1982).

TFR

An overall equation for estimating the TFR directly from the proximate determinants is obtained by substituting Equations (11), (13), and (14) in Equation (19). Assuming an absence of induced abortion and a use-effectiveness of $e = 0.85$, this equation simplifies to

$$\text{TFR} = 15.3 \times C_m \times (1 - 1.08 \times u \times 0.85) \times 20/(18.5 + i) \qquad (22)$$

Using this equation, Table 4.6 presents estimates of TFR for selected values of C_m, u, and i covering the normal observed ranges for these vari-

Table 4.6
**MODEL ESTIMATES OF THE TOTAL FERTILITY RATE FOR DIFFERENT
DURATIONS OF POSTPARTUM INFECUNDABILITY, DIFFERENT VALUES OF
C_m AND DIFFERENT LEVELS OF CONTRACEPTIVE PREVALENCE[a]**

Prevalence of	Duration of postpartum infecundability (months)				
contraceptive use	3.0	6.0	12.0	18.0	24.0
			$C_m = 0.45$		
0.0	6.9	5.6	4.5	3.8	3.2
0.2	5.6	4.6	3.7	3.1	2.7
0.4	4.4	3.6	2.9	2.4	2.1
0.6	3.1	2.5	2.0	1.7	1.5
0.8	1.8	1.5	1.2	1.0	0.9
			$C_m = 0.65$		
0.0	9.2	8.1	6.5	5.4	4.7
0.2	7.5	6.6	5.3	4.4	3.8
0.4	5.9	5.1	4.1	3.4	3.0
0.6	4.2	3.6	2.9	2.4	2.1
0.8	2.5	2.2	1.7	1.4	1.2
			$C_m = 0.85$		
0.0	12.1	10.6	8.5	7.1	6.1
0.2	9.9	8.7	7.0	5.8	5.0
0.4	7.7	6.7	5.4	4.5	3.9
0.6	5.4	4.8	3.8	3.2	2.8
0.8	3.2	2.8	2.3	1.9	1.6

[a] Source: Equation (22).

ables. Each of these proximate determinants has a strong influence on the TFR. Changing C_m from 0.85 to 0.45 lowers the TFR by almost the same proportion as is obtained by increasing postpartum infecundability from 3 to 24 months, but both these effects are smaller than the fertility-reducing impact of a change in prevalence from $u = 0$ to $u = 0.8$. As was the case for marital fertility, a given level of the TFR can be obtained by a variety of combinations of C_m, u, and i, and populations with the same TFRs will only rarely have the same proximate variables. It should be noted that not all combinations of the proximate determinants are observed with equal frequency. Developed countries typically have lower values of C_m combined with high levels of contraceptive prevalence and short durations of postpartum infecundability. The opposite picture is usually found in developing countries (i.e., high C_m and i values, and low us).

The foregoing estimates of TN, TM, and TFR were based on the Equations (17), (18), and (19), which assumed that the only measures available for the estimation of fertility levels are the indexes or the proximate determinants from which they are derived. In practice, a good estimate of the TFR or the TM is often readily obtained in a population where the necessary data to calculate the indexes are available. In that case, more accurate estimates of the different fertility levels can be made.[5] For example, if the indexes C_m, C_c, C_a, and C_i, as well as the TFR, are known in population, then the TF would be equal to

$$TF = TFR/(C_m \times C_c \times C_a \times C_i) \tag{23}$$

This equation gives an exact estimate of the TF only if the variables required for the calculation of TF are accurate. This is rarely the case in practice, and the equation may consequently produce an estimate with a significant error. Large errors in the indexes or in the TFR are easily detected with Equation (23). For example, if the resulting TF is 20, which is well outside the normal range of 13 to 17, one can be virtually certain that an error has been in the estimation of one of the variables on the right-hand side of Equation (23).

SUMMARY

This chapter presents a simple but comprehensive model for the relationship between the proximate determinants and a set of aggregate fertility measures, including the TFR and the TM. Four of the proximate variables—marriage, contraception, induced abortion, and postpartum infecundability—are considered the principal determinants of fertility, whereas the remaining three proximate variables—natural fecundability, spontaneous intrauterine mortality, and permanent sterility—are treated as generally much less important determinants. A test of the model with data from 41 developing, developed, and historical populations indicated that the four principal proximate determinants explained 96% of the variance in the observed TFRs of these populations, thus confirming the general validity of the model and the hypotheses about the operation of the reproductive process incorporated in it. In the last section, the effects of variations in the proximate variables on levels of overall, marital, and natural fertility were examined with the model. This analysis demonstrated that each of the principal proximate variables can have a large impact on fertility and that any given level of fertility can be obtained by a variety of combinations of the proximate determinants. As a consequence, populations with the same TFR do not necessarily, and in fact only rarely, have the same set of proximate determinants. It was also noted that marital fertility may temporarily rise during an early phase of the demographic transition if the fertility-enhancing

[5] Equations for estimating fertility levels from the indexes and at last one other fertility rate are:

for TF: $TF = TFR/(C_m \times C_c \times C_a \times C_i) = TM/(C_c \times C_a \times C_i) = TN/C_i$;

for TN: $TN = TFR/(C_m \times C_c \times C_a) = TM/(C_c \times C_a) = TF \times C_i$;

for TM: $TM = TFR/C_m = TN \times C_c \times C_a = TF \times C_i \times C_c \times C_a$;

for TFR: $TFR = TM \times C_m = TN \times C_m \times C_c \times C_a = TF \times C_m \times C_c \times C_a \times C_i$.

effect of a decline in breastfeeding or postpartum abstinence is not offset by a sufficiently rapid increase in the practice of contraception or induced abortion.

APPENDIX: AN EQUATION FOR ESTIMATING C_c

Define the following age-specific variables for a population of married women:

a = age, in single years.
$f(a)$ = proportion that is fecund (i.e., nonsterile).
$p(a)$ = proportion of fecund women that attempts to prevent pregnancies by contracepting. These women will be called "contraceptors."
$u(a)$ = proportion that currently uses contraception.
$v(a)$ = proportion of contraceptors that currently uses contraception, that is, the proportion not accidentally pregnant or in postpartum amenorrhea.
$e(a)$ = contraceptive use-effectiveness.
$N(a)$ = mean duration of the nonsusceptible segment of the birth interval, consisting of pregnancy and postpartum infecundable periods.
$C(a)$ = mean duration of the susceptible ovulatory segment of the birth interval in the absence of contraception.
$F(a)$ = fertility rate of all married women (births per woman per year).
$F_n(a)$ = natural fertility rate of all married women.
$F_c(a)$ = fertility rate of contraceptors.
$F_a(a)$ = fertility rate of fecund noncontraceptors.

If it is assumed that contraceptors are always fecund, the population can be divided into three subpopulations: the contraceptors, the fecund noncontraceptors, and the sterile women. The fertility rate of all (married) women equals the weighted average of the fertility rate of contraceptors and noncontraceptors.

$$F(a) = p(a)f(a) F_c(a) + [1 - p(a)]f(a) F_a(a) \tag{1}$$

If one further assumes that fecund women are homogeneous with respect to their fecundity characteristics, then

$$F_a(a) = \frac{1}{N(a) + C(a)} \tag{2}$$

$$F_c(a) = \frac{1}{N(a) + \dfrac{C(a)}{1 - e(a)}} \tag{3}$$

$$F_n(a) = \frac{f(a)}{N(a) + C(a)} \tag{4}$$

The homogeneity assumption can be relaxed by allowing heterogeneity within each of the subgroups of contraceptors and noncontraceptors, but on average the two groups have to be equal in their fecundity characteristics. In either case, the exchange of women between the two groups is allowed if the proportion $p(a)$ is not affected.

Within the subpopulation of contraceptors, a small proportion of women is in the nonsusceptible state because accidental pregnancies occur. If all other contraceptors are using contraception, then the proportion of contraceptors that is currently using equals:

$$v(a) = \frac{\dfrac{C(a)}{1 - e(a)}}{N(a) + \dfrac{C(a)}{1 - e(a)}} \tag{5}$$

so that

$$u(a) = p(a)\,f(a)\,\frac{\dfrac{C(a)}{1 - e(a)}}{N(a) + \dfrac{C(a)}{1 - e(a)}} \tag{6}$$

Equation (6) can be rearranged as

$$p(a) = u(a)\,\frac{N(a) + \dfrac{C(a)}{1 - e(a)}}{f(a)\,\dfrac{C(a)}{1 - e(a)}} \tag{7}$$

Substitution of Equations (2), (3), and (7) in (1) results in:

$$F(a) = F_n(a)\left[1 - \frac{u(a)e(a)}{f(a)}\right] \tag{8}$$

If more than one method of contraception is employed, $u(a)$ equals the total use of all methods and $e(a)$ equals the weighted average effectiveness (weights given by the proportions using different methods).

The foregoing derivation assumes that couples know their fecundity status and that only fecund couples will use contraception. In reality, some sterile couples believe that they are still fecund. It is easily demonstrated that Equation (8) is also valid if $f(a)$ measures the proportion of women that believes that they are fecund, provided that the proportion using contraception among the actually fecund women is the same as among the women who believe they are fecund. (The above equations also assume no overlap of contraceptive use with postpartum infecundability. The error caused by this assumption is small and offset by a selection for higher than average fecundability among contraceptors [Bongaarts, 1982]).

The expression in brackets in Equation (8) gives the age-specific index of contraception. The aggregate index is obtained as follows.

The TM is found by summing $F(a)$ over all age groups in the reproductive period (35 years between ages 15 and 50):

$$TM = \Sigma\, F(a)$$

$$= \Sigma\, F_n(a)\left[1 - \frac{u(a)e(a)}{f(a)} \right] \qquad (9)$$

$$= TN - \Sigma\, F_a(a)u(a)e(a)$$

where $F_a(a)$ represents the age-specific natural marital fertility rate among fecund women. Equation (9) can be simplified further because the variable $F_a(a)$ declines only modestly with age, and the product $u(a)\,e(a)$ has an inverted U shape, first rising and then declining with increasing age. Consequently, with good approximation,

$$TM = TN - \tfrac{1}{35}F_a\,\Sigma\, u(a)e(a) = TN - F_a e u \qquad (10)$$

with the averages F_a, e, and u defined as

$$F_a = \Sigma\, F_a(a) \qquad (11)$$

$$e = \Sigma\, e(a)\, u(a)/u \qquad (12)$$

$$u = \tfrac{1}{35}\,\Sigma\, u(a) \qquad (13)$$

That Equation (10) provides a good approximation for TM can be confirmed by substituting standard schedules for $F_n(a)$, $f(a)$, $u(a)$, and $e(a)$ in Equations (10) and (9). In addition, u can in practice be approximated by the proportion currently using among all married women aged 15–49. If one further defines

$$s = \Sigma\, \frac{F_n(a)}{f(a)} \bigg/ \Sigma\, F_n(a) \qquad (14)$$

then Equation (10) becomes

$$TM = TN(1 - seu) = TN \times C_c \qquad (15)$$

An estimate of $s = 1.08$ for developing countries was obtained by substituting the standard Coale-Trussel schedule for $F_n(a)$ (Coale and Trussell 1973) and by using for $f(a)$ the empirical schedule of age-specific proportions of women who believe they are fecund proposed by Nortman (1980). (In an earlier study (Bongaarts 1978), the coefficient s was estimated to equal 1.18 on the inaccurate assumption that all women know their fecundity status and that all contraceptive users are fecund).

REFERENCES

Bongaarts, J. (1978), "A Framework for Analyzing the Proximate Determinants of Fertility," *Population and Development Review*, 4, 1, 105–132.

Bongaarts, J. (1982), "The Fertility Inhibiting Effects of the Intermediate Fertility Variables," *Studies in Family Planning,* 13, 6/7, 179–189.

Bongaarts, J. (1982), "The Concept of Potential Fertility in the Evaluation of the Fertility Impact of Family Planning Programs." Paper presented at the Third Expert Group Meeting on Methods of Measuring the Impact of Family Planning Programs on Fertility, United Nations, Geneva.

Bongaarts, J. and S. Kirmeyer (1982), "Estimating the Impact of Contraceptive Prevalence on Fertility: Aggregate and Age-Specific Versions of a Model," in the *Role of Surveys in the Analysis of Family Planning Programs,* A. Hermalin and B. Entwisle, Eds., Ordina, Liege.

Cho, L. (1973), "The Demographic Situation in the Republic of Korea," Papers of the East-West Institute, No. 29.

Coale, A. J., "Factors Associated with the Development of Low Fertility: An Historic Summary," *Proceedings of the World Population Conference,* United Nations, New York, 1967.

Coale, A. J. and T. J. Trussell (1974), "Model Fertility Schedules: Variations in the Age Structure of childbearing in Human Populations," *Population Index, 40,* 195–258.

Knodel, J. (1982), "Natural Fertility: Age Patterns, Level Trends," in *Determinants of Fertility in Developing Countries:* A Summary of Knowledge, National Academy of Sciences, Washington, D.C. (forthcoming).

Laing, J. (1978), "Estimating the Effects of Contraceptive Use on Fertility," *Studies in Family Planning, 9,* 6, 150–175.

Leridon, H. (1977), *Human Fertility: The Basic Components,* University of Chicago Press, Chicago.

Menken, J., J. Trussell, K. Ford, and W. F. Pratt (1979), "Experience with Contraceptive Methods in Developed Countries," in *Contraception: Science, Technology and Applications,* Washington, National Academy of Sciences.

Nortman, D. (1980), "Sterilization and the Birth Rate," *Studies in Family Planning, 11,* 9–10, 286–300.

Potter, R. (1972), "Births Averted by Induced Abortion," *Theoretical Population Biology, 3,* 1, 69–86.

Su, L. P., and L. P. Chow, (1976), "Induced Abortion and Contraceptive Practice: An Experience in Taiwan," *Studies in Family Planning 7, 8* 24–230.

5

Applications of an Aggregate
Fertility Model

An aggregate model for the relationship between the fertility and its proximate determinants was described and tested in the preceding chapter. To
illustrate how this model may be used to gain insight into the operation of the
proximate determinants or to solve specific problems, we will summarize in
this chapter a set of applications dealing with a variety of topics.

APPLICATION 1:
THE TRANSITION IN THE PROXIMATE DETERMINANTS

As a population moves through the transition from natural to controlled
fertility there is, by definition, an increase in deliberate marital fertility control. This control is exerted primarily through a rise in contraceptive use, but
in a number of populations the practice of induced abortion plays a major
role. Accompanying the transition in the deliberate control of marital fertility
are transitions in the other principal proximate determinants—marriage and
postpartum infecundability. As a consequence of these trends in the proximate determinants, important changes take place in the levels of natural
marital fertility, marital fertility, and overall fertility.

To examine changes in these fertility measures over the course of the
transition, it is unfortunately not possible to rely on time trends in individual

populations because the necessary data are lacking. Instead, a comparative analysis will be made here of contemporary populations at different points in the transition. The result will be an outline of a fairly typical "synthetic" transition from the fertility behavior found in contemporary developing countries to that currently observed in developed countries. To provide a clearer picture of the trends in the proximate determinants, populations are divided into four groups according to the level of fertility, giving an approximate indication of the transition phase.

Phase of transition in fertility	Total fertility rate
I	over 6.0
II	4.5–6.0
III	3.0–4.5
IV	less than 3.0

The fertility of most populations in Phase I is close to natural, whereas populations in Phase IV have completed most or all of the fertility transition.

Estimates of the proximate determinants, the indexes C_m, C_c, C_a, and C_i, and the TN, TM, and TFR of groups of populations in each of the four transition phases are obtained by averaging the data of 31 developing and developed countries from Tables 4.2 and 4.3. The results are presented in Table 5.1 and Figure 5.1. (All estimates in Table 5.1 are subject to large sampling errors because of small numbers of populations included in each transition phase.) The TN rises from 9.93 to 14.23 births per woman between the first and last phase of the transition, as the consequence of a shortening of the mean duratio of postpartum infecundability from 12.9 to 3.0 months. Despite the large increase in TN, the TM declines from 9.08 to 3.80 during the transition. The reason is clearly a large rise in the contraceptive prevalence—from 0.10 to 0.69, accompanied by an increase in contraceptive use-effectiveness from 0.85 to 0.94. Induced abortion plays, on average, a minor or negligible role except in the last two phases of the transition when its effect becomes significant. Interestingly, the decline in marital fertility during the first three phases is quite modest, as the increase in the practice of contraception only barely manages to compénsate for the fertility-enhancing impact of a shortening of the duration of postpartum infecundability. Finally, the TFR changes from 7.03 to 2.06 during the transition, due to the reduction in marital fertility but also because C_m declines from 0.78 to 0.55. This decline in the proportion of women married is largely the result of a rise in the mean age at marriage (see Chapter 3).

Table 5.1

AVERAGES OF MEASURES OF THE PROXIMATE DETERMINANTS, THE INDEXES AND THE OVERALL, MARITAL AND NATURAL MARITAL FERTILITY RATES FOR GROUPS OF POPULATIONS IN DIFFERENT PHASES OF A SYNTHETIC TRANSITION[a]

	Phase of fertility transitions			
	I	II	III	IV
Prevalence of contraceptive use (u)	0.10	0.35	0.40	0.69
Use-effectiveness of contraception (e)	0.85	0.85	0.86	0.94
Total induced abortion rate (TA)	0.0	0.0	0.38	0.46
Postpartum infecundability (i)	12.9	7.6	8.5	3.0
Index of marriage (C_m)	0.780	0.627	0.551	0.550
Index of contraception (C_c)	0.912	0.682	0.630	0.301
Index of induced abortion (C_a)	1.000	1.000	0.961	0.887
Index of postpartum infecundability (C_i)	0.649	0.780	0.763	0.930
Total fertility rate (TFR)	7.03	5.03	3.88	2.06
Total marital fertility rate (TM)	9.08	8.08	7.05	3.80
Total natural marital fertility rate (TN) [b]	9.93	11.93	11.67	14.23
Number of countries included	7	11	4	9

[a] Source: Tables 4.2 and 4.3.

[b] Estimated as $15.3 \times C_i$.

In sum, this outline of the transition in the different fertility measures indicates that a typical transition from natural to controlled fertility is accompanied by a shortening of postpartum infecundability, a large increase in contraceptive use, and a decline in the proportion married. It should be emphasized that this pattern is based on a comparison of contemporary populations at different stages in the transition. Actual transitions over time in developing countries probably resemble this pattern quite closely, but the transitions in historical European countries are different in one respect. Instead of a reduction in the proportion married, these historical populations typically have experienced a decline of the mean age at marriage and a rise in the proportion of women married (Watkins 1981).

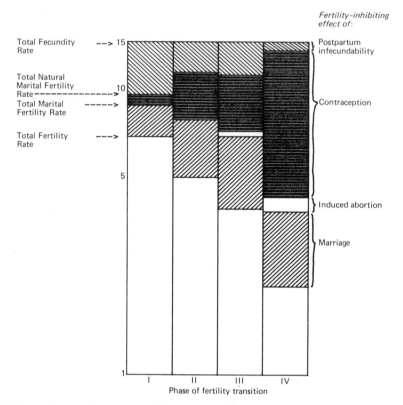

FIGURE 5.1. Estimated average total natural marital fertility rates, total marital fertility rates, and total fertility rates of countries in different phases of the fertility transition.

APPLICATION 2:
DECOMPOSITION OF A CHANGE IN FERTILITY

It was concluded earlier that any change in a population's level of fertility is necessarily caused by a change in one or more of the proximate determinants. We will now present a set of equations that allow the quantification of the contribution made by each proximate determinant to a given change in fertility.

A Summary of the Decomposition Procedure

The decomposition of a trend in the TFR is based on the following equation, which links the TFR to the fertility-inhibiting effects of the four principal proximate variables (marriage, contraception, induced abortion, and postpartum infecundability) measured by the indexes C_m, C_c, C_a, and C_i, and to TF (see Chapter 4 for details):

$$\text{TFR} = C_m \times C_c \times C_a \times C_i \times \text{TF} \tag{1}$$

Let Year 1 and Year 2 represent, respectively, the first and last year of the time period for which a decomposition is desired. With a change in the TFR from TFR1 in Year 1 to TFR2 in Year 2 and with simultaneous changes in the indexes from C_m1 to C_m2, from C_c1 to C_c2, from C_a1 to C_a2, from C_i1 to C_i2, and from TF1 to TF2 between Year 1 and Year 2, the ratio TFR2/TFR1 can be expressed as

$$\frac{\text{TFR2}}{\text{TFR1}} = \frac{C_m2}{C_m1} \times \frac{C_c2}{C_c1} \times \frac{C_a2}{C_a1} \times \frac{C_i2}{C_i1} \times \frac{\text{TF2}}{\text{TF1}} \tag{2}$$

Defining further

$P_f = \text{TFR2/TFR1} - 1$
= proportional change in TFR between Year 1 and Year 2 $\tag{3}$

$P_m = C_m2/C_m1 - 1$
= proportional change in TFR due to a change in the index of marriage $\tag{4}$

$P_c = C_c2/C_c1 - 1$
= proportional change in TFR due to a change in the index of contraception $\tag{5}$

$P_a = C_a2/C_a1 - 1$
= proportional change in TFR due to a change in the index of induced abortion $\tag{6}$

$P_i = C_i2/C_i1 - 1$
= proportional change in TFR due to a change in the index of postpartum infecundability $\tag{7}$

$P_r = \text{TF2/TF1} - 1$
= proportional change in TFR due to changes in the remaining proximate variables—natural fecundability, spontaneous intra-uterine mortality, and permanent sterility $\tag{8}$

Equation (2) can now be rearranged as

$$P_f = P_m + P_c + P_a + P_i + P_r + I \tag{9}$$

where I represents an interaction factor.[1] This equation simply states that a given proportional change in the TFR between Year 1 and Year 2 equals the sum of the proportional fertility changes due to the different proximate de-

---

[1] Rearranging Equations (3), (4), (5), (6), (7), and (8), and substitution of the results in Equation (2) yields

terminants plus an interaction term. (This interaction factor is a complex function of P_m, P_c, P_a, P_i, and P_r, which will not be presented here. I can of course be estimated simply by subtracting the sum of P_m, P_c, P_a, P_i and P_r from P_f. In general, I is small if the P values are small and have mixed positive and negative signs.) Equation (9) can easily be turned into a decomposition equation for the absolute decline in the TFR, TFR2 − TFR1, by multiplying both sides by TFR1 (see Footnote 1 for equations).

An Illustration of the Decomposition Procedure

The decomposition of the proportional change in the TFR into the components P_m, P_c, P_a, P_i, and P_r requires the calculation of the P values from the indexes C_m, C_c, C_a, and C_i. The estimation of these indexes, in turn, requires measures of the proximate determinants. This procedure will now be illustrated with a decomposition of the decline in the TFR of Korea during the 1960s. The required measures of the proximate determinants for 1960 and 1970 are presented in the upper panel of Table 5.2. From these variables, the indexes and TF given in the bottom panel of Table 5.2 are calculated (see Chapter 4 for equations). Finally the estimates of the indexes and TF are used to calculate the different P factors presented in the first column of Table 5.3. These results indicate that the TFR decline of 35.2% between 1960 and 1970 can be decomposed into a 19.4% decline due to a decrease in the proportion of women married, a 20.6% decline due to an increase in contraceptive practice, a 12.4% decline due to an increase in the practice of induced abortion, and a 17.9% increase due to shortening of the duration of postpartum infecundability. The remaining proximate variables together contribute only 1.9%, and the interaction factor equals 1.2%. In the second column of Table 5.3, the decomposition results are standardized to add to 100%, and in the last column the absolute change in the TFR of 2.16 births per woman between 1960 and 1970 is decomposed into the contributions made by the various proximate variables.

An alternative way to summarize the contributions made by the principal proximate determinants to a change in the TFR is presented in Figure 5.2. It

---

$$1 + P_f = (1 + P_m) \times (1 + P_c) \times (1 + P_a) \times (1 + P_i) \times (1 + P_r)$$
$$= 1 + P_m + P_c + P_a + P_i + P_r + I$$

where I consists of all second and higher order products of P factors. Subtracting 1 from both sides of this equation produces Equation (9).

Multiplication of both sides of Equation (9) by TFR1 results in the following equation for the decomposition of the absolute change in the TFR:

$$\text{TFR2} - \text{TFR1} = \text{TFR1} \times (P_m + P_c + P_a + P_i + P_r + I)$$

Table 5.2

ESTIMATES OF SELECTED FERTILITY MEASURES, PROXIMATE DETERMINANTS AND INDEXES OF PROXIMATE DETERMINANTS FOR KOREA 1960 AND 1970[a]

	1960	1970
Total fertility rate (TFR)	6.13	3.97
Total marital fertility rate (TM)	8.57	6.85
Proportion currently using contraception (u)	0.03	0.24
Contraceptive use-effectiveness (e)	0.85	0.89
Total abortion rate (TA)	0.52	1.50
Duration of postpartum infecundability (i)	17.4	11.9
Index of marriage (C_m)	0.72	0.58
Index of contraception (C_c)	0.97	0.77
Index of induced abortion (C_a)	0.97	0.85
Index of postpartum infecundability (C_i)	0.56	0.66
Total fecundity rate (TF)	16.2	15.9

[a] Source: Bongaarts (1978), Tables 4.2 and 4.3 and equations (10), (11), (13), (14) and (23) in Chapter 4.

Table 5.3

DECOMPOSITION OF THE CHANGE IN THE KOREAN TOTAL FERTILITY RATE BETWEEN 1960 AND 1970

Factors responsible for fertility change	Percentage[a] of change in TFR	Distribution of percentage of change in TFR	Absolute change in TFR
Proportion of women married	−19.4	−55.1	−1.19
Contraceptive practice	−20.6	−58.5	−1.26
Practice of induced abortion	−12.4	−35.2	−0.76
Duration of postpartum infecundability	+17.9	+50.9	+1.10
Other proximate determinants	− 1.9	− 5.4	−0.12
Interaction	+ 1.2	+ 3.4	+0.07
Total	−35.2	100.0	−2.16

[a] Calculated with Equations (3) − (9) from data in Table 5.2.

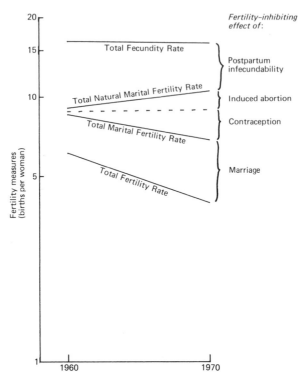

FIGURE 5.2. Changes in measures of fertility and fertility-inhibiting effects of proximate variables from Korea (1960–1970).

plots the trends in the TFR, the TM, the TN, and the TF.[2] The differences between the successive levels of fertility are due to the fertility-inhibiting effects of the corresponding proximate determinants (see Figure 5.2). (A meaningful comparison of these differences requires a logarithmic transformation). As expected, there is a substantial increase in natural marital fertility due to a shortening of the duration of postpartum infecundability, but TM and TFR decline as a result of the increase in the practice of contraception and induced abortion as well as a decline in the proportion married.

A Decomposition of a Change in the Crude Birth Rate

The decomposition procedure for the TFR can easily be extended to also allow the decomposition of a change in the crude birth rate (CBR).

---

[2] TM, TN, and TF are calculated from

$$TM = TFR/C_m$$
$$TN = TFR/(C_m \times C_c \times C_a)$$
$$TF = TFR/(C_m \times C_c \times C_a \times C_i)$$

The CBR is linked to its proximate determinants by the following equation, derived from Equation (9):

$$CBR = S \times C_m \times C_c \times C_a \times C_i \times TF \qquad (10)$$

where S is an age–sex composition factor calculated as

$$S = CBR/TFR \qquad (11)$$

Variations in S are caused by changes in the population's age–sex structure. If we define further

$$P_b = CBR2/CBR1 - 1$$
$$= \text{proportional change in the CBR between} \qquad (12)$$
$$\text{Years 1 and 2}$$

$$P_s = S2/S1 - 1$$
$$= \text{proportional change in CBR due to a change in the} \qquad (13)$$
$$\text{age–sex composition.}$$

then it can be shown that

$$P_b = P_s + P_m + P_c + P_a + P_i + P_r + I \qquad (14)$$

where P_m, P_c, P_a, P_i, and P_r have the same values as in Equation (9).

In Korea, the CBR declined by 33%, from 43.3 to 29.0, during the 1960s (Cho 1973). The decomposition of this decline, presented in Table 5.4, shows that, in addition to the contributions made by the various proximate deter-

Table 5.4
DECOMPOSITION OF CHANGE IN THE KOREAN CRUDE BIRTH RATE BETWEEN 1960 AND 1970

Factors responsible for CBR change	Percentage of change in CBR	Distribution of percentage of change in CBR	Absolute change in CBR
Age–sex structure	+ 3.4	+10.3	+1.47
Proportion of women married	−19.4	−58.8	−8.41
Contraceptive practice	−20.6	−62.4	−8.92
Practice of induced abortion	−12.4	−37.6	−5.38
Duration of postpartum infecundability	+17.9	+54.2	+7.75
Other proximate determinants	− 1.9	− 5.8	−0.83
Interaction	0.0	0.0	0.0
Total	−33.0	100.0	−14.3

[a] Source: Table 5.3 and Equations (11) – (14).

minants, the age–sex composition changed slightly, contributing a 3.4% increase to the CBR.

APPLICATION 3: SOCIOECONOMIC DIFFERENTIALS IN MARITAL FERTILITY

In an earlier discussion of socioeconomic differentials in marital fertility, it was concluded that one would expect lower than average marital fertility among women in higher socioeconomic groups. Available data indicated that women living in urban areas and those with higher education or with husbands in nonagricultural occupations had generally lower marital fertility. There were however a number of exceptions. For example, in Pakistan marital fertility in urban areas was higher than in rural areas. To explain this and similar anomalous findings, it is necessary to analyze the socioeconomic differentials in the proximate determinants of marital fertility.

The principal determinants of marital fertility are contraceptive prevalence and the duration of postpartum infecundability if no induced abortion is practiced. Observed socioeconomic differentials in these proximate determinants are usually in the direction one would expect from their trends during the early phases of the fertility transition. That is, among urban and educated women, contraceptive prevalence is above average, and the duration of postpartum infecundability is below the population average (Jain and Bongaarts 1981, Lesthaeghe, Shah and Page 1981). These urban–rural differentials are also found in the case of Pakistan (1975), which will be used here for the purpose of illustration. The measurements in the upper panel of Table 5.5 show that contraceptive prevalence among urban women was .15 compared to only .02 among rural women, and the durations of postpartum infecundability were 11.9 and 15.8, respectively, for urban and rural areas. Yet the marital fertility difference is not in the expected direction: the TM in urban areas is 9.48 births per woman compared with only 8.85 for rural women. An explanation for this finding is found in the lower panel of Table 5.5, which summarizes a decomposition of the urban–rural marital fertility difference with the procedure described in the preceding section. According to these decomposition results, the fertility-inhibiting effect of -11.8% due to higher contraceptive use in urban areas was not sufficient to offset the fertility-enhancing effect of 12.9% due to a shorter duration of postpartum infecundability among urban women. Furthermore, differentials in the other proximate determinants added 7.6% to urban marital fertility (this is perhaps caused by a greater incidence of seasonal spousal separations in rural areas), and the interaction factor equaled -1.5%. As a consequence, urban marital fertility was 7.1% higher than rural marital fertility.

Table 5.5
SELECTED REPRODUCTIVE MEASURES FOR URBAN AND RURAL PAKISTAN IN 1975, AND DECOMPOSITION OF RURAL-URBAN FERTILITY DIFFERENCE

Selected reproductive measures	Rural	Urban
Total marital fertility rate (TM)	8.85	9.48
Proportion currently using contraception (u)	0.02	0.15
Duration of postpartum infecundability (i)	15.8	11.9
Index of contraception (C_c)	0.982	0.866
Index of postpartum infecundability (C_i)	0.583	0.658
Total fecundity rate (TF)	15.46	16.64

Factors responsible for rural-urban differential in marital fertility	Percentage of difference in marital fertility
Contraceptive practice	−11.8
Postpartum infecundability	+12.9
Other proximate determinants	+ 7.6
Interaction	− 1.6
Total rural urban difference	7.1

Source: The total marital fertility rates (TMs) by place of residence in Pakistan were estimated from data in Table 4.2 and Table 3.1. Residence specific contraceptive prevalence and duration of postpartum amenorrhea were taken from Lesthaeghe et al., 1981. Contraceptive use-effectiveness of rural and urban areas were assumed to be equal to the national average of 0.83 given in Chapter 4. The decomposition results are obtained with a procedure similar to the one described in Application 2. Instead of referring to two points in time, 1 and 2 now refer to rural and urban populations, respectively, and instead of decomposing a difference in the TFR a decomposition of TM is given in Table 5.5. Let P_{mf} be the proportional difference in TM between rural and urban areas, then $p_{mf} = P_c + P_a + P_i + P_r + I$ where the P values are estimated with Equations (5) − (8).

In general, the higher contraceptive prevalence levels and shorter durations of postpartum amenorrhea are found among women in higher socioeconomic status groups. Whether these differentials in the proximate determinants lead to higher or lower marital fertility depends entirely on the size of the differences. The fertility-inhibiting effect of higher contraceptive use is usually sufficient to compensate for the decline in postpartum infecundability, but a modest differential in contraceptive prevalence combined with a relatively large difference in postpartum infecundability will result in increased marital fertility in the higher socioeconomic status groups.

APPLICATION 4:
AN AGE-SPECIFIC FERTILITY MODEL

An age-specific model for the relationship between age-specific fertility rates and their proximate determinants is obtained by a straightforward extension of the aggregate model discussed thus far. Instead of the total rates, TFR, TM, TN, and TF, their age-specific counterparts (measured in births per 1000 women per year) are introduced:

$AFR(a)$ = age-specific fertility rates (a = age of woman)
$AM(a)$ = age-specific marital fertility rates
$AN(a)$ = age-specific natural marital fertility rates
$AF(a)$ = age-specific fecundity rates

Similarly, the aggregate indexes, C_m, C_c, C_a, and C_i, are replaced by the age-specific indexes $C_m(a)$, $C_c(a)$, $C_a(a)$, and $C_i(a)$, which measure the fertility-inhibiting effects of the four principal proximate determinants in each age group. Estimates of these indexes are made from age-specific measures of the proximate determinants.[3]

As in the aggregate model, the age-specific fertility rates can be expressed as the product of the indexes and the fecundity rates:

$$AFR(a) = C_m(a) \times C_c(a) \times C_a(a) \times C_i(a) \times AF(a) \qquad (15)$$

---

[3] Define the following age-specific variables for a population of women of reproductive age ($AFR(a)$, $AM(a)$, $AN(a)$, $AF(a)$ are defined in the text):

a = age
$m(a)$ = proportions currently married or in stable sexual union
$u(a)$ = proportion currently using contraception among married women
$e(a)$ = use-effectiveness of contraception
$f(a)$ = proportion currently believed to be fecund
$A(a)$ = induced abortion rate (abortions per 1000 women per year)
$i(a)$ = duration of postpartum infecundability

The age-specific indexes are calculated from the following equations, which are based on the corresponding equations for the aggregate indexes derived in Chapter 4:

$$C_m(a) = m(a)$$
$$C_c(a) = 1 - u(a) \times e(a)/f(a)$$
$$C_a(a) = \frac{AFR(a)}{AFR(a) + 0.4 \times (1 + u(a)) \times A(a)}$$
$$C_i(a) = \frac{20}{18.5 + i(a)}$$

$$AM(a) = C_c(a) \times C_a(a) \times C_i(a) \times AF(a) \qquad (16)$$

$$AN(a) = C_i(a) \times AF(a) \qquad (17)$$

A thorough analysis of the age-specific model is beyond the scope of this chapter, but one example of an application will be presented here. In this application model, estimates will be made of the $AM(a)$s in the first two phases of the synthetic fertility transition outlined earlier and summarized in Table 5.1 and Figure 5.1. Between Phase I and Phase II of this transition, the average TM declined slightly as the result of an increase in average contraceptive prevalence from 10 to 35%, combined with a decline in the aver-

---

The age-specific proximate variables $u(a)$, $e(a)$, $f(a)$, $i(a)$, and the age-specific fecundity rates $AF(a)$ used in Application 4 were based on the following standard age patterns:

	$u(a)$	$e(a)$	$f(a)$	$AF(a)$
15–19	.194	—	—	(511)
20–24	.295	.61	.98	682
25–29	.375	.80	.97	641
30–34	.423	.90	.96	549
35–39	.418	.91	.89	414
40–45	.335	.98	.75	205
45–49	.211	.91	.48	59

—$u(a)$: This standard age pattern was obtained by averaging the age-specific proportions currently using contraception in 26 populations (Bongaarts and Kirmeyer 1982). The average proportion contracepting in all age groups is .322; to arrive at higher or lower prevalence levels, the standard pattern is proportionately inflated or deflated.

—$e(a)$: The standard pattern of use effectiveness was estimated by Bongaarts and Kirmeyer (1982) with a regression analysis similar to the one used in Application 5. The higher levels of use effectiveness among older women are the consequence of higher motivation and lower degree of chance-taking as well as of greater reliance on the more effectiveness contraceptive methods including sterilization.

—$f(a)$: The values of $f(a)$ were taken from Nortman (1980). It should be emphasized that the $f(a)$ values are estimates of the proportions believed to be fecund. These are larger than the actual proportions fecund or nonsterile because some women (couples) do not realize that they have become sterile.

—$i(a)$: As noted in the text, the duration of postpartum infecundability can be assumed constant, if combined with the same equation for $C_i(a)$, without great loss in accuracy.

—$AF(a)$: The same regression analysis that produced the standard pattern of use-effectiveness levels also yielded estimates of the age-specific fecundity rates (Bongaarts and Kirmeyer 1982). This pattern has been multiplied here by a factor 1.004 to ensure that the sum of the age-specific fecundity rates add to 15.3. As is the case for the age-specific marital and natural marital fertility rates, $AF(15–19)$ is set equal to $0.75 \times AF(20–24)$. (See Footnote 1 in Chapter 4.) Bongaarts and Kirmeyer (1982) have shown that the shape of the age pattern of $AF(a)$ is very similar to that of the standard Coale–Trussell natural fertility pattern, although the level of the former is higher than that of the latter.

age duration of postpartum infecundability from 12.9 to 7.6 months. To arrive at the corresponding model age-patterns for contraceptive prevalence and postpartum infecundability given in the first two columns of Table 5.6, it is assumed that the prevalence rates follow the standard pattern proposed by Bongaarts and Kirmeyer (1982) and that the duration of postpartum infecundability is constant. Although postpartum infecundability in reality rises

Table 5.6
AGE SPECIFIC CONTRACEPTIVE PREVALENCE RATES, DURATIONS OF POSTPARTUM INFECUNDABILITY AND FECUNDITY RATES, AND MODEL ESTIMATES OF AGE SPECIFIC MARITAL FERTILITY RATES FOR PHASES I AND II OF A SYNTHETIC FERTILITY TRANSITION[a]

Age	Proportion currently contracepting $[u(a)]$	Duration of postpartum infecundability $[i(a)]$	Age specific fecundity rate $[AF(a)]$	Model estimates of age specific marital fertility rate $[AM(a)]$
		Phase I of fertility transition		
15–19	0.06	12.9	(511)[b]	(307)[b]
20–24	0.09	12.9	682	409
25–29	0.12	12.9	641	366
30–34	0.13	12.9	549	306
35–39	0.13	12.9	414	230
40–44	0.10	12.9	205	117
45–49	0.07	12.9	59	35
Total	0.10	12.9	15.3	8.9
		Phase II of fertility transition		
15–19	0.21	7.6	(511)[b]	(309)[b]
20–24	0.32	7.6	682	412
25–29	0.41	7.6	641	317
30–34	0.46	7.6	549	233
35–39	0.45	7.6	414	177
40–44	0.36	7.6	205	97
45–49	0.23	7.6	59	35
Total	0.35	7.6	15.3	7.9

[a] Source: See text and Footnote 3.
[b] Estimated as 75% of rate in age group 20–24.

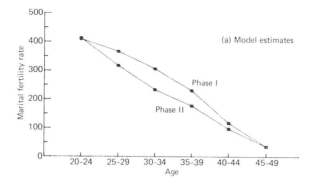

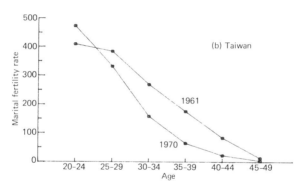

FIGURE 5.3.   Model estimated age-specific marital fertility rates for phases I and II of a synthetic demographic transition and age-specific marital fertility rates for Taiwan, 1961 and 1970.

slightly with age, the other components of birth intervals increase also, so that the fertility-inhibiting impact of postpartum infecundability changes very little with age. It is, therefore, simpler and more convenient to use the same equation for $C_i(a)$ in all age groups and to assume the duration of postpartum infecundability to be age invariant.

The indexes $C_c(a)$ and $C_i(a)$ can now be calculated from the age-specific measures of contraceptive prevalence and postpartum infecundability, and multiplication of the standard AF(a)s by $C_c(a)$ and $C_i(a)$ yields the AM(a)s in the last column of Table 5.6 (see Footnote 3 for details). Summing the AM(a)s ($\times 5$) gives TMs of 8.9 and 7.9 for Phase I and II, respectively. These values are slightly lower than those reported in Table 5.1 because the estimates in that table were averages for heterogeneous groups of populations. The model estimates in Table 5.6 are made for a homogeneous population and no allowance is made for heterogeneity.

These model age-patterns of marital fertility for the first two phases of the synthetic fertility transition are plotted in Figure 5.3a. Interestingly, marital fertility as estimated by the model does not decline uniformly at all ages between Phases I and II. The fertility of married women in age group 20–24 is projected to rise from 409 to 412 births per 1000 women. The cause of this trend in AM(20–24) is not difficult to pinpoint: The relatively small increase in contraceptive prevalence combined with a relatively low level of use-effectiveness in this age group produced a relatively small increase in the fertility-inhibiting effect of contraception that was insufficient to compensate for the effect of a decline in postpartum infecundability. The opposite is the case in the other age groups. Although this lack of uniformity in the change in marital fertility is somewhat unexpected, it has actually been observed in a number of populations. For example, the AM(a)s of Taiwan, plotted in Figure 5.3b, show a rise for age group 20–24 from 409 in 1961 to 473 in 1970, whereas overall marital fertility declined over the same period of time (Freedman, Hermalin, and Sun 1972). Similar patterns of change in marital fertility have also been found in the early phases of the demographic transition of historical populations (Knodel 1982). Of course, in many other populations marital fertility declines continuously over time at all ages. Whether and to what extent marital fertility rises temporarily in some age groups depends on the competing effects of the proximate variables. The balance of the effects of contraceptive prevalence and the duration of postpartum infecundability is especially important as the trend in the model patterns indicated, but other factors may also play a role. For example, the observed increase in marital fertility of 20- to 24-year-old women in Taiwan during the 1960s may, in part, be due to a slight rise in the TF or to a relatively more rapid decline in the duration of postpartum infecundability among younger women.

APPLICATION 5: THE EMPIRICAL RELATIONSHIP BETWEEN FERTILITY AND CONTRACEPTIVE PREVALENCE

It has been noted repeatedly in the literature that a high degree of correlation exists between the fertility and contraceptive prevalence levels of contemporary populations (Berelson 1974, Nortman 1980). Perhaps the most widely used relationship between a measure of fertility and contraceptive prevalence is based on the regression of the CBR on prevalence (u). Nortman (1980), for example, estimates the following regression equation from data for 32 developing countries:

$$
\begin{aligned}
\text{CBR} &= 46.9 - 42.0 \times u \\
&= 46.9 \times (1 - 0.90 \times u) \qquad R^2 = .91
\end{aligned}
\tag{18}
$$

This equation confirms that there is a high correlation between u and CBR. However, it is not at all clear that u, in fact, causes a change in fertility of the magnitude indicated by this equation. The CBR is influenced by factors other than contraception, such as the population's age structure, the marriage pattern, the duration of postpartum infecundability, and the incidence of induced abortion. It is necessary to control the influence of these factors before one can arrive at the correct relationship between fertility and contraceptive prevalence.

To accomplish this, regression analysis will be used here to examine the relationships between prevalence and a number of different measures of fertility, at each step removing one of the confounding variables. The data for the 22 developing countries used in this exercise are taken from the upper panel of Table 4.2. (Korea and the developed countries are excluded because the analysis is limited to populations with presumably insignificant levels of induced abortion.)

Contraceptive Prevalence and the TFR

The effects of the age structure of the population are removed by taking the TFR as the measure of fertility instead of the CBR. The close association between the TFR and contraceptive prevalence, u, is summarized in the regression equation

$$TFR = 7.3 - 6.4 \times u$$
$$= 7.3 \times (1 - 0.88 \times u) \qquad R^2 = 0.72 \qquad (19)$$

The intercept 7.3 represents the expected level of natural fertility, that is, fertility in the absence of contraception (and induced abortion). The slope of the regression line equal to 6.4 gives an estimate of the decline in the TFR associated with increaes in u and the relative slope equal to 0.88 gives the proportional decline. For example, if 50% of married women of reproductive age are current users of contraception ($u = 0.5$) then the TFR is expected to be $6.4 \times 0.5 = 3.2$ below the natural level of 7.3, a reduction of 44% ($0.88 \times 0.5 = 0.44$). The relative slope in Equation (19) is virtually the same as in Equation (18),—0.88 versus 0.90—suggesting that, on average, the age structure of the population does not have an important disturbing effect on the regressions of the CBR on contraceptive prevalence.

Prevalence and the TM

To examine the effect of contraceptive use on fertility free of the influence of the marriage pattern, the TM is used as the fertility indicator. The relationship between the TM and prevalence, u, is given in the following regression equation:

$$TM = 9.5 - 4.8 \times u$$
$$= 9.5 \times (1 - 0.51 \times u) \qquad (R^2 = 0.40) \qquad (20)$$

A comparison of this equation with the regression for the total fertility rate shows two differences: a higher intercept and a lower slope (see also Figure 5.4). The higher intercept is to be expected because in all countries the TFR is lower than TM, which is not affected by the fertility-inhibiting effect of the marriage pattern. The lower relative slope indicates that an increase in prevalence has relatively less impact on marital fertility than on the TFR. This finding is explained by the correlation between contraceptive prevalence and proportions married among women of reproductive age. Populations with high levels of contraceptive use tend to have relatively high ages at first marriage and more marital disruption. As a consequence, Equation (19) contains a bias for a steeper slope that is eliminated in Equation (20).

Prevalence and Marital Fertility in the Absence of Postpartum Infecundability

Although the effect of differences in marriage patterns is controlled in Equation (20), it is not free of the confounding influence of population differences in the duration of postpartum infecundability induced by lactation or postpartum abstinence. To remedy this shortcoming, an adjusted total marital fertility rate (TMA) is calculated. The TMA is equal to the TM in the absence of postpartum infecundability and is estimated as: $TMA = TM/C_i$. Regressing TMA on u yields:

$$TMA = 15.3 - 13.7 \times u$$
$$= 15.3 \times (1 - 0.90 \times u) \qquad R^2 = 0.92 \qquad (21)$$

The intercept of 15.3 in this regression is much higher than in Equation (20), indicating the powerful effect of postpartum infecundability on natural fertility. The relative slope is also much higher. This is to be expected from the negative correlation between contraceptive prevalence and lactation duration. Countries with high prevalence levels typically have the shortest breastfeeding intervals. As a consequence, the difference between TMA and TM decreases with increasing contraceptive-use levels (see Figure 5.4). Equation (21) finally gives what may be considered the unbiased fertility impact of contraceptive prevalence because the influence of the age structure, marriage pattern, and breastfeeding duration have been removed. (No correction is made for the other proximate determinants because it was shown earlier that they have, on average, little effect on fertility trends and differentials). Interestingly, the relative slope of Equation (21) is virtually the same as in Equation 19. This implies that, with increasing contraceptive

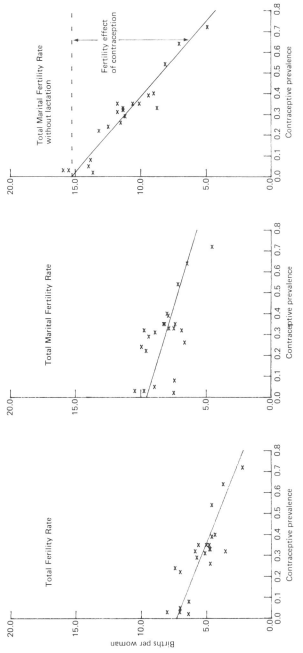

FIGURE 5.4. Regression lines with the total fertility rate, the total marital fertility rate, and the total marital fertility rate without lactation as dependent variables and contraceptive prevalence as the independent variable. Data points represent 22 developing countries.

prevalence levels, the fertility effects of shortened postpartum infecundability are, on average, almost exactly compensated by the smaller proportions married.

A partial explanation for the empirical results summarized in Equations (19), (20), and (21) has already been provided. The difference between the regression lines for TFR and TM are the result of the fertility-inhibiting effect of the marriage pattern, and the difference between TM and TMA is attributable to the influence of postpartum infecundability. According to the aggregate fertility model, Equation (21) can now be interpreted as the product of the TF and C_c. The multiplication factor $(1 - 0.9 \times u)$ on the right side of Equation (21) represents the fertility-inhibiting effect of contraception, which according to the theoretical model should be equal to $C_c = 1 - 1.08 \times e \times u$. Setting the relative slopes of regression line (21) equal to the theoretical slope $(0.90 = 1.08 \times e)$ yields a regression estimate of the average use-effectiveness of contraception $e = 0.83$ $(= 0.90/1.08)$. This estimate can be compared with an independently obtained estimate of 0.85 for the average contraceptive use-effectiveness of the 22 contemporary developing populations with no induced abortion in the upper panel of Table 4.2. The close agreement between these two estimates indicates that the empirical findings regarding the fertility impact of contraceptive prevalence and effectiveness are consistent with the theoretical fertility effect estimated from $C_c = 1 - 1.08 \times u \times e$, thus confirming the validity of the latter.

An important result of the last regression is that it provides an independent estimate of the TF. The intercept of the regression line represented by Equation (21) equals 15.3 births per woman. This is an estimate of the TN in the absence of postpartum infecundability, which has been defined as the TF. In the preceding chapter, an approximate value of TF = 15 was obtained with a highly simplified calculation. The present estimate of TF = 15.3 is more accurate and it has been used in all analyses in this as well as in the preceding chapter.

APPLICATION 6: PROJECTED FERTILITY TRENDS ASSOCIATED WITH CHANGES IN CONTRACEPTIVE PRACTICE

Let TFR1 and TFR2 be the TFRs, in respectively, Year 1 (the present) and Year 2 (a year in the future), and let the corresponding levels of contraceptive prevalence and use-effectiveness be $u1$ and $e1$, and $u2$ and $e2$, respectively. The objective now is to estimate the level of TFR2 if contraceptive practice changes between Year 1 and Year 2.

The problem is not difficult to solve if one assumes that the indexes for all other proximate determinants remain constant. That is, the marriage pattern, the duration of postpartum infecundability, the incidence of induced abor-

Table 5.7

PROJECTED TOTAL FERTILITY RATES FOR INDONESIA IN 1985, ESTIMATED FROM ASSUMED TREND IN CONTRACEPTIVE PREVALENCE AND USE-EFFECTIVENESS[a]

Assumed contraceptive prevalence in 1985 (u2)	Assumed contraceptive use-effectiveness in 1985 (e2)	Projected total fertility rate in 1985 (TFR2)
0.30	0.87	4.46
0.35	0.87	4.17
0.40	0.87	3.87
0.45	0.87	3.58
0.50	0.87	3.29

[a] Source: Equation (22); for 1976: TFR1 = 4.69, u1 = 0.26 and e1 = 0.87.

tion, and the TF are taken to be the same in Year 1 and Year 2. In that case it can be shown that[4]

$$TFR2 = TFR1 \times (1 - 1.08 \times u2 \times e2)/(1 - 1.08 \times u1 \times e1) \quad (22)$$

The results of an application of this equation in Indonesia are given in Table 5.7. The TFR in Indonesia in 1985 is projected for different levels of contraceptive prevalence in that year. For simplicity, the contraceptive use-effectiveness is assumed to remain at the 1976 level of 0.87. In 1976, the TFR in Indonesia is estimated to have been 4.69 and contraceptive prevalence was 0.26 (Bongaarts and Kirmeyer 1982). The projection results in Table 5.7 show that the decline in fertility varies directly with the increase in contraceptive prevalence. For example, if prevalence rises to 0.40, the TFR would be 3.87 in 1985, whereas a prevalence of 0.50 would be required to reach a TFR of 3.29.

The validity of Equation (22) and the accuracy of the projected fertility levels in Table 5.7 depend on the assumption that the indexes for all proximate variables other than contraception remain constant. This is not the case in general. It is possible to estimate changes in fertility if all proximate determinants change with Equation (2), but this would require detailed data that are often not available. Fortunately the much simpler Equation (22) is also valid if changes in the other proximate determinants compensate one another. It was demonstrated in the previous application that, on average, the positive fertility effect of a shortening of postpartum infecundability is offset by the negative fertility effect of a decline in the proportion of married women. As a conse-

[4] Equation (22) is derived from Equation (2) with substitution of $C_m1 = C_m2$, $C_a1 = C_a2$, $C_i1 = C_i2$, TF1 = TF2, $C_c1 = (1 - 1.08 \times u1 \times e1)$ and $C_c2 = (1 - 1.08 \times u2 \times e2)$. The change in contraceptive practice is assumed not to affect C_m or C_a.

quence, Equation (22) can be used even if the marriage pattern and the duration of postpartum infecundability change, provided that these factors on balance have a negligible effect on the fertility trend. The robustness of Equation (22) is further enhanced by the fact that in the short run, say up to a few years, the marriage pattern or the duration of postpartum infecundability usually do not change substantially.

The application of Equation (22) for the estimation of future levels of fertility would of course not be accurate if the incidence of induced abortion increased rapidly or if the TF changed substantially. However, this is usually not a problem because the incidence of induced abortion is negligible in many populations and the TF rarely varies significantly over time.

APPLICATION 7: CONTRACEPTIVE PREVALENCE LEVELS REQUIRED TO REACH A FERTILITY TARGET

Governments of a substantial number of developing countries make efforts to limit fertility by encouraging contraceptive use (Nortman and Hofstatter 1980). Often specific fertility goals are set for future years. Administrators of family planning programs are then faced with the question of what level of contraceptive prevalence and effectiveness to aim for in order to reach the fertility target.

The answer to this question is provided by the following equation, if the indexes for the other proximate determinants are constant or compensate each other[5]:

$$u2 \times e2 = (1 - TFR2 \times (1 - 1.08 \times u1 \times e1)/TFR1)/1.08 \qquad (23)$$

The 1 and 2 refer to the present and a given year in the future, as in the previous application. This equation demonstrates that a specific fertility goal TFR2 can be reached with a variety of combinations of contraceptive prevalence and effectiveness as long as the product $u2 \times e2$ is equal to level estimated by Equation (23). If methods with low use-effectiveness are expected to be used in Year 2, then a higher prevalence level will be required to meet the target. On the other hand, fewer contraceptive users would be needed if a switch to more effective methods took place. This is illustrated in Table 5.8, which presents estimates of the contraceptive use and effectiveness levels needed to obtain TFRs of 4.0, 3.5, and 3.0 in Indonesia in a given future year. For example, Indonesia's TFR in say the year 1985 would be 3.0 if the proportion of contracepting women were raised to 53% with a use-effectiveness of 0.9, but a prevalence of only 48% would be needed if use-effectiveness could be raised to 1.0 by relying strictly on sterilization. Although it is in principle possible to project contraceptive requirements for

---

[5] Equation (23) is obtained by rearranging Equation (22). It is again assumed that a change in contraceptive practice does not affect Cm or Ca.

Table 5.8
**MODEL ESTIMATES OF CONTRACEPTIVE PREVALENCE AND USE-EFFECTIVENESS
REQUIRED TO REACH FUTURE FERTILITY TARGETS IN INDONESIA**

Future fertility target (TFR2)	Contraceptive use-effectiveness in target year (e2)	Contraceptive prevalence required to reach fertility target (u2)
4.0	0.85	0.39
4.0	0.90	0.37
4.0	0.95	0.35
4.0	1.00	0.33
3.5	0.85	0.48
3.5	0.90	0.45
3.5	0.95	0.43
3.5	1.00	0.40
3.0	0.85	0.56
3.0	0.90	0.53
3.0	0.95	0.50
3.0	1.00	0.48

[a] Source: Equation (23) (it is assumed that the other proximate determinants are constant or compensate each other; $TFR1 = 4.69$, $u1 = 0.26$ and $e1 = 0.87$).

lower levels of fertility in later years, this is not done here because the assumption that the indexes for the other proximate determinants are constant or compensate each other is likely to become less realistic as time progresses.

SUMMARY

The aggregate fertility model described in Chapter 4 can be used to gain insights into a variety of theoretical and practical issues concerning the relationship between fertility and the proximate determinants. In this chapter, seven separate applications of the model are summarized. In the first, estimates are made of the trends in the principal proximate determinants during a "synthetic" transition from the fertility behavior found in contemporary developing countries to that currently observed in developed countries. The second described a decomposition procedure that allows the quantification of the contribution made by each proximate determinant to an observed fertility change between two points in time. This procedure is used in the third application to demonstrate how socioeconomic differentials in the proximate determinants can explain unexpected differentials in marital fertility. The fourth presents an age-specific elaboration of the aggregate fertility model. Presented next is an analysis of the empirical relationship between contraceptive prevalence levels and different fertility measures. In the sixth application, future levels of the total fertility rate are projected based on estimated trends in contraceptive practice. The chapter concludes with a brief description and application of an equation for estimating the levels of contraceptive prevalence and use-effectiveness required to reach a prescribed fertility target.

REFERENCES

Berelson, B. (1974), *World Population: Status Report,* Reports on Population/Family Planning, No. 15, The Population Council, New York.

Bongaarts, J. (1978), "A Framework for Analyzing the Proximate Determinants of Fertility," *Population and Development Review, 4* 1, 105–132.

Bongaarts, J. (1982), "The Fertility Inhibiting Effects of the Intermediate Fertility Variables," *Studies in Family Planning,* 13, 6/7, 179–189.

Bongaarts, J. and S. Kirmeyer (1982), "Estimating the Impact of Contraceptive Prevalence on Fertility: Aggregate and Age-Specific Versions of a Model," in *The Role of Surveys in the Analysis of Family Planning Programs,* A. Hermalin and B. Entwisle, Eds., Ordina, Liege.

Cho, L. (1973), "The Demographic Situation in the Republic of Korea," Papers of the East-West Institute, No. 29.

Freedman, R., A. Hermalin and T. H. Sun (1972), "Fertility Trends in Taiwan: 1961–1970," *Population Index, 38,* 2, 141–165.

Jain, A. K. and J. Bongaarts (1981), "Breastfeeding: Patterns, Correlates, and Fertility Effects," *Studies in Family Planning, 12,* 3, 79–108.

Knodel, J. (1982), "Natural Fertility: Age Patterns, Level Trends," in *Determinants of Fertility in Developing Countries: A Summary of Knowledge,* National Academy of Sciences, Washington, D.C. (forthcoming).

Lesthaeghe, R. J., I. H. Shah and H. J. Page (1981), "Compensating Changes in Intermediate Fertility Variables and the Onset of Marital Fertility Transition," in *Proceedings of IUSSP General Conference, Manila,* Ordina, Liege, 1981.

Nortman, D. (1980), "Sterilization and the Birth Rate," *Studies in Family Planning, 11,* 9–10, 286–300.

Nortman, D. and E. Hofstatter (1980), *Population and Family Planning Programs: A Compendium of Data through 1978,* A Population Council Fact Book, 10th Ed., The Population Council, New York.

Watkins, S. C. (1981), "Regional Patterns of Nuptiality in Europe 1870–1960," *Population Studies, 35,* 2 (July), 199–216.

6

A Macrosimulation Model and Applications to Fecundity and Natural Fertility

INTRODUCTION

Chapters 2–5 are concerned with average completed family size and its determination by a short list of proximate factors. The chapters focus on the ways that total fertility rates respond as particular intervening variables, or subsets thereof are changed. Throughout, a deterministic aggregative approach has been taken. Though the models employed in Chaper 2–5 are far from simple, still they are modest enough in their data demands so that requisite information from a number of nations can be brought to bear and genuine comparative analysis thereby achieved.

The objectives of the next four chapters require that more complicated reproductive models be utilized. One focus of interest is the variation of fertility among individual couples and, more particularly, the variation attributable to chance factors. Conceptive waits vary randomly as do lengths of postpartum anovulation and outcomes of pregnancy. Moreover these different sources of chance variation operate synergistically and, at least in the absence of deliberate fertility control efforts, accumulate over birth intervals. In real life the contributions of chance factors to variation in family size and birth intervals is confounded with variations resultant from systematic

differences among couples. However with the aid of an appropriate reproductive model, that component of variation owing to randomness can be
isolated. By making the hypothetical cohort of couples under study homogeneous with respect to fecundity, age at marriage, and fertility goals, any
variation of fertility remaining is properly ascribed to chance factors.

A second and perhaps more important focus of interest is the relative
difficulty of different fertility goals and some of the conditions raising or
lowering this difficulty. Three types of goal are distinguished: family size,
birth spacing, and sex composition or sequencing of children. A proper reproductive model permits the creation of simulated cohorts of couples. In
such a cohort sharing a common family-size goal, the dispersion of final
parities around the targeted number of children measures the difficulty of
attaining that goal. In similar simulated cohorts, the dispersion of birth times
around a targeted duration gauges the attainability of a spacing goal. Deviations of realized sex compositions measure the accessibility of a particular
sex compositional goal. And for all three types of goals, the significant
characteristics of the cohort may be altered to see how the difficulty of goal
achievement rises or falls.

A closely related interest is the theoretical limits of fertility control. How
far can the inherent variability of the components of fertility be suppressed in
the service of particular family goals? Compared this time are cohorts alike
in such aspects as fecundity and fertility goals, but pursuing different control
strategies to achieve them. For example, one may ask what level of contraceptive effectiveness and how much back-up by induced abortion is required to realize specified standards of family-size control. Or what decision
rule about when to interrupt contraception serves best to minimize the scatter of birth times around a target duration. Or again, how much less efficient
at achieving a desired sex composition is a particular strategy that demands
fewer diagnoses of fetal sex and fewer corrective abortions on average than a
second strategy? By means of reproductive models, experimentation on
hypothetical cohorts of couples becomes an expedient matter; whereas such
experimentation on real couples would be quite unfeasible, not to say un-
ethical.

A fourth focus of interest is the compatibility of different fertility goals. A
case is made that commitment to a sex compositional goal tends to weaken
both spacing and family-size control. On the other hand, except in special
circumstances, pursuit of spacing goals hardly comprises the control of child
number; only to minor extents do birth-spacing goals exacerbate subfertility or facilitate avoidance of excess births.

Not surprisingly, pursuit of these interests calls for more complicated
reproductive models than employed in Chapters 2–5. As part of their standard output, they must yield fertility variation at the individual couple level.
They must be able to incorporate fertility goals and the control strategies

associated with them. As always, the interest of their results depends on the realism of their assumptions. Input requirements are high. Because of these data exigencies, the contexts for all applications will be confined to the United States (early mid-1970s) and rural Bangladesh (roughly the same period), two of the very few settings for which the requisite input data can be marshalled.

In Chapters 6, 7, and 8, heavy reliance is placed on the macrosimulation model REPMOD. Not only has its standard version been updated, but several variants have been elaborated for particular analyses. Because of these developments and because of its practical interest as a general purpose and economical macrosimulation, REPMOD is believed to be worth describing in some detail. Two more analytical and specialized reproductive models are employed in Chapters 8 and 9, but their algebra is not taken any further than in the articles originally reporting them.

In the division of labor among the next four chapters, Chapter 6 considers variation in family size when fertility control efforts are absent. Chapter 7 examines final numbers of children when control efforts are present. Chapter 8 addresses birth-spacing control. Chapter 9 appraises the only currently effective approach, namely midtrimester diagnoses of fetal sex and corrective abortion, to controlling sex composition and sequencing of children.

Turning specifically to Chapter 6, the longest section titled REPMOD presents an updated version of the computer model to be principally relied on. Specific technical issues are pursued in footnotes. For perspective, this description is preceded by a review of the three main types of reproductive models capable of expressing fertility variation among couples as a function of systematic differences among them together with the operation of chance factors. To justify the reliance being placed on REPMOD, a successful validation of it at the time of its first publication is also briefly reviewed. The general reader may want to skip over, or at least reserve for a second reading, the initial sections that have to do with technical aspects.

The ensuing sections, of a substantive nature, explore variation in total fertility, first under fecundity conditions and then under those of natural fertility. *Fecundity*, defined as natural fertility freed from the inhibitions of lactational infecundability and delayed or interrupted marriage, represents a hypothetical state of affairs. The natural fertility population is patterned after rural Bangladesh. In both cases, tremendous variation in final family sizes is deduced for couples whose marriages remain intact until the end of the reproductive period. It is of interest to apportion these large variations of final parity among three sources: differences among couples in reproductive length (i.e., intervals from marriage to onset of natural sterility), differences among couples in level of natural fecundability, and chance factors. It is demonstrated that the last of the three, stochastic variation, plays a highly significant role.

REPRODUCTIVE MODELS

Three classes of reproductive models may be distinguished.

Mathematical Models

Mathematical models consist of equations linking fertility events directly to their determinants. Fairly realistic, but highly aggregated, models of this type have been described in the previous chapters. Such mathematical models can yield reasonable estimates of mean fertility, but when one wants to look at fertility variation, then additional simplifying assumptions have to be made with attendant losses of realism. For example, one common class of reproductive model, the Markov renewal process, presupposes three strong assumptions: *homogeneity* (all couples share the same parameter values), *stationarity* (parameters do not change with age or marriage duration), and an unlimited reproductive period, to avoid truncation effects. The most exhaustive treatment of these models is offered by Sheps and Menken (1973). An outline of standard results obtainable from these renewal processes is given in Potter (1969). Although unrealistic for the second half of the reproductive period when parameter values are changing rapidly, the renewal-type models have proven useful for investigating the dynamics of pregnancy and birth intervals in the first few years of marriage. Such a model is employed in Chapter 8 to explore strategies for controlling the interval between first and second births. Another mathematical model is utilized in Chapter 9 to investigate strategies of sex preselection.

Macrosimulation Models

Macrosimulation models typically have a mathematical basis consisting of a set of equations that cannot be solved analytically. However, by programming these equations on a computer, numerical solutions may be calculated. Macromodels are deterministic because the rates at which reproductive events occur are exactly determined by the assumed probabilities of transitions between reproductive states (e.g., pregnant, amenorrheic, fecundable, sterile). They are "expected value" models mimicking the dispersions and central tendencies of birth intervals and final parities that might be recorded in a very large population. Freedom from sampling fluctuations makes their results well suited for "if, then" demonstrations, that is, for showing fertility responses when one or more intermediate variables are changed in specified ways. Because macrosimulations allow changes in the transition probabilities as a function of age or duration, they do not require the simplifying assumption of either stationarity or an unlimited reproductive period. Nor does homogeneity have to be assumed inasmuch as the experience of several homogeneous subcohorts, weighted appropriately, may be merged. Thus, when fertility distributions are of interest as well as fertility means, macrosimulations allow more realism than do mathematical models.

A number of macromodels for simulating human reproduction have been developed: for example, the FERMOD series (Ford, 1976, Potter, Sakoda, and Feinberg 1968, and Potter and Sakoda, 1966, and 1967,), ACCOFERT I and II (Potter, 1971 and 1972), and REPMOD (Bongaarts, 1977). The last is favored over FERMOD on account of its up-to-dateness and superior economy of operation and it is favored over ACCOFERT because it encompasses entire reproductive careers instead of just events following attainment of desired family size. Several improvements have been made to REPMOD since its publication in 1977. The revised version is described in the next section and applications of it made to fecundity and natural fertility in later sections.

Microsimulation Models

By means of this technique, also called "Monte Carlo simulation," histories of reproductive events are simulated for one woman at a time. For each female partner, the successive reproductive states entered or the intervals between events are partly determined by a series of random numbers with values between 0 and 1 generated in the computer. Repeating this process many times produces a collection of reproductive histories for which as much detailage as desired may be retained. In effect, one cumulates a databank. Not only can a much more detailed output be realized by the Monte Carlo approach, but a much more complicated structure of determinants in terms of interdependencies among parameters and between-couple heterogeneities with respect to particular parameters can be achieved than is feasible with a macrosimulation model.

Examples of existing microsimulation models are those developed by Barrett (1969), Bodmer and Jacquard (1968), Holmberg (1970, 1972), Jacquard (1967), Ridley and Sheps (1966), and Venkatacharya (1971).[1] However, the superior versatility of this type of model has not meant a commensurate increase in realism because of the lack of field data to guide the intricate assumptions operationally feasible. Moreover, Monte Carlo results are subject to sampling fluctuations. Two simulations under identical assumptions never produce identical results. To reduce this random error, one may increase sample size, but this adds to computer costs. In the chapters that

[1] Most Monte Carlo models of human reproduction have simulated birth, marriage, or acceptor cohorts. An exception is the well-documented microsimulation model POPSIM that represents period populations. A special version of POPSIM, encompassing the full spectrum of family building components, is described in Lachenbruch, Sheps, and Sorant (1973).

follow, macrosimulation is favored over microsimulation for the sake of results free from sampling fluctuation and greater economy of operation. It is believed that REPMOD commands enough realism for interesting results.

REPMOD

Outline of the Model

Two diagrams provide overviews of REPMOD. The state transition diagram in Figure 6.1 presents the sequence of reproductive states through which women progress from birth to end of childbearing, in the absence of sterility or marital disruption by divorce or widowhood. Note that the set of states depicted in Figure 6.1 are precisely the states implied by Figure 1.1 when provision is being made for intrauterine deaths. Her own birth finds every woman in the unmarried state. While in this state she is at risk of marrying. The probability of first marriage at each month of age is derived from a first marriage distribution. Upon marriage, the woman enters into the fecundable state, putting her at risk of conception. This monthly risk may be reduced to a low level by practice of contraception. After a random number of months, she becomes pregnant. A pregnancy ends either in a live birth or a fetal loss (spontaneous or induced). All pregnancy terminations after the conception month other than live births are treated as intrauterine deaths, whereas fertilized ova that disappear before the menstrual period is missed are disregarded. Contingent on fetal loss, the woman occupies a state of temporary nonsusceptibility for the duration of the interrupted pregnancy plus the associated postpregnancy infecundable period and then returns to

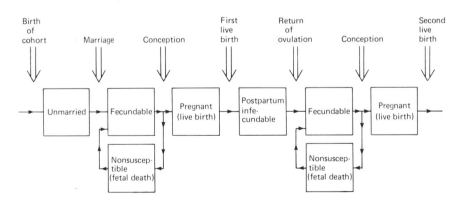

FIGURE 6.1. State transition diagram.

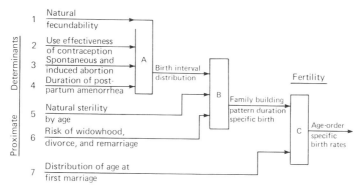

FIGURE 6.2. Relationships between the inputs or independent variables and the outputs.

the fecundable state. Given a live birth, the 9 months of full-term pregnancy are followed by a postpartum anovulatory period. The end of this period marks the beginning of a new fecundable interval.

The preceding progression through reproductive states is continued until interrupted by permanent sterility or marital disruption. With childbearing outside of marriage not allowed in the model, the only way a divorced or widowed woman can return to the reproductive process is through remarriage.

Figure 6.2 outlines the relationships between the proximate fertility determinants serving as inputs or independent variables in REPMOD and the fertility outputs or dependent variables. The first four proximate fertility determinants shape birth interval distributions and can vary with age, duration of marriage, or parity (level of interaction A in Figure 6.2). Natural fecundability and the use and effectiveness of contraception govern the mean duration of the waiting time to conception. Induced or spontaneous abortion prevents a conception from ending in a live birth. The mean duration of the postpartum anovulatory period varies according to the pregnancy outcome and, in the case of a live birth, may be prolonged by breastfeeding. At level of interaction B, family-building patterns or duration-specific birth rates are determined by a sequence of birth intervals, commencing with marriage. The childbearing process proceeds until it is interrupted by the onset of permanent sterility, widowhood, or divorce. Finally, at interaction level C, the fertility pattern of the entire cohort exists as a combination of the duration-specific birth rates of the different first-marriage cohorts. The sizes of these cohorts is dictated by the distribution of first marriages by age.

The principal outputs of the model are the age and the age-order-specific birth rates of the entire cohort. If marriage age is made constant, so that a one-to-one relationship exists between age of wife and marriage duration, then distributions of duration from marriage to births of specified orders can also be generated along with duration or duration-order-specific birth rates.

Specification of REPMOD's Basic Operation

The most primitive version of REPMOD involves the following simplifications: (a) The cohort is homogeneous (i.e., all women share the same parameter values and therefore are biologically indistinguishable); (b) there is no deliberate birth control; (c) The birth interval determinants—natural fecundability, risk of spontaneous abortion, and mean duration of postpartum anovulation—are constant over age; and (d) there is no disruption of marriages by divorce or widowhood.

In the next section each of these restrictions will be removed, resulting in what may be called the "standard version" of REPMOD. For purposes of Chapters 7 and 8, even the standard version of REPMOD will have to be elaborated, the description of these elaborations being deferred until Chapter 7.

The differential equations embodying the rudimentary version of REPMOD require that the distribution of waiting times in each of the following reproductive states be specified.

UNMARRIED STATE

The first marriage distribution, giving the proportion of the cohort leaving the unmarried state by month of age, is determined by the marriage model of Coale and McNeil (1972). Required is the specification of three parameters: (a) initial age at first marriage; (b) mean age at first marriage; and (c) proportion of the birth cohort ever marrying.[2] Alternatively, an arbitrary first-

---

[2] Discussed in Coale (1977) is the standard frequency distribution of first marriages formally derived in Coale and McNeil (1972),

$$g(x) = .1946\,e^{-0.174(x-6.06)-e^{-0.2881(x-6.06)}}$$

where x measures time in years from the initial age at marriage. The mean duration generated by $g(x)$ equals 11.36. This standard distribution $g(x)$ may be turned into a general marriage function $g(a)$ of age a by introducing three parameters:

a_0 = initial age at marriage
k = time scale factor
C = proportion ever marrying.

By use of substitution $x = (a - a_0)/k$,

marriage distribution, including the special case of a constant marriage age, may be substituted.

FECUNDABLE STATE

Following previous studies (Potter and Parker 1964, Sheps 1964), the waiting-time distribution in this state is represented by a geometric distribution that is wholly governed by one parameter, natural fecundability.

PREGNANT STATE BEFORE A LIVE BIRTH

The duration of a pregnancy ending in a live birth is taken as 9 months.

POSTPARTUM ANOVULATORY STATE

Following Barrett (1969), the waiting time in this state is assumed to be that Pascal distribution that is equivalent to the convolution of two geometric variates.[3] Whereas one of its two parameters equals the integer 2, the other is derived from the estimated mean duration of the postpartum anovulation period.

NONSUSCEPTIBLE PERIOD ASSOCIATED WITH A SPONTANEOUS ABORTION

In the case of a spontaneous abortion, the waiting time from conception to the end of postabortion anovulation is treated as geometrically distributed with parameter $g = .40$. The proportion of all pregnancies that ends in a spontaneous abortion is controlled by parameter a, the risk of spontaneous abortion.

The differential equations embodying the mathematics of REPMOD are predicated on the preceding waiting-time distributions. The only additional

---

$$g(a) = \frac{.1946C}{k}\ e^{(-0.174/k)(a-a_0-6.06k)-e^R}$$

$$R = -2.881(a - a_0 - 6.06k)/k.$$

Let $\bar{a}$ denote the mean age generated by function $g(a)$. From $k = (\bar{a} - a_0)/11.36, \bar{a} = 11.36k + a_0$.

[3] The waiting time in this state is assumed to be the sum of two geometrically distributed subintervals governed by a common parameter h. This parameter is chosen to give an expected value, $1/h + 1/h$, equalling the mean of the observed distribution being fitted. The corresponding variance is $2(1 - h)/h^2$. When mean length is small, near the minimum length of 2.0, then h is near 1.0 and necessarily the variance $2(1 - h)/h^2$ is small. The distribution is very close to one proposed by Barrett (1969), which has been shown to fit well either distributions of brief anovulation, reflective of absent or brief breastfeeding, or else intermediate length anovulation averaging 9–12 months consequent upon longer lactation.

function that must be specified in order to implement the primitive version of REPMOD is the incidence of sterility by age. For this function the age pattern of sterility estimated by Henry (1965) is used although any other pattern could as easily be specified. To introduce sterility into the model, it would be possible to subject women to the risk of sterility at every age and in each of the reproductive states, but it is much simpler to complete the simulation of the entire sequence of reproductive events without sterility and eliminate afterward those events that would not have occurred if sterility were, in fact, present. For example, if the age-specific birth rate in the absence of sterility is $b(t)$ and the proportion of all women that are sterile by age t (in months) is $s(t)$, then the recorded age-specific fertility rate is simply $b(t)[1 - s(t - 9)]$.[4]

The Standard Version of REPMOD

For greater flexibility and realism, four extensions are made to the core rendition of REPMOD.

HETEROGENEITY WITH RESPECT TO NATURAL FECUNDABILITY

It is assumed that the entire cohort is divisible into a number of homogeneous subcohorts. Natural fecundability differs among subcohorts according to a given fecundability distribution. A set of reproductive events is calculated for each subcohort separately, and to find the rates and distributions of the total cohort the weighted average of all subcohorts is taken.

Earlier research (Bongaarts 1975), based on several historical series of European ancestry, indicated for the interval from marriage to first birth that, although the mean of fecundability varies considerably from sample to sample, its coefficient of variation varies in a much narrower range (.53–.63 in six series investigated). Furthermore, when this heterogeneity of fecundability is partitioned into a persistent and a transitory component, the former explains from slightly more than one-half to two-thirds of the total. In order

---

[4] The age pattern of sterility is read into the computer program as a set of proportions nonsterile N_x at exact age x in years. The values adopted starting with N_{19} and running to N_{50} are .98, .97, .97, .97, .96, .96, .95, .95, .94, .94, .93, .92, .91, .90, .89, .87, .85, .82, .79, .76, .72, .68, .63, .57, .49, .40, .31, .23, .15, .09, .05, and .00. For ages $x < 19$, $N_x = .98$, consistent with a 2% minimum primary sterility rate. It is assumed that births during month t are rendered impossible only if sterility has occurred by month $t - 9$. Although in REPMOD a sterility reduction factor is applied to births monthly, that factor is treated as a constant over each year of age. Women aged x at last birthday average $x + 0.5$ years, and 9 months subtracted from that mid-age yields $x - .25$ in years. Hence the most appropriate sterility proportion for reducing births among women aged x at last birth is that characterizing women aged exactly $x - .25$, which is approximated by $N_x^* = .75N_x + .25N_{x-1}$. Thus the set N_x, taken directly from Henry's analysis, constitute input, but they are transformed into the set N_x^* before application.

that REPMOD incorporate this component of persistent fecundability, a standard distribution is defined as three equally weighted subcohorts having $0.5f_n$, $1.0f_n$, and $1.5f_n$ as their natural fecundabilities, yielding a coefficient of variation of .41.

BIRTH CONTROL

During the married, nonsterile childbearing years, women are assumed to progress through three phases. First, they are noncontraceptors; then upon reaching the desired number of births they become contraceptors; and, finally, a proportion of the contraceptors may resort to induced abortion to prevent further unwanted births.

A contraceptive regime is specified by (*a*) the distribution of the number of desired births in the cohort; and (*b*) the contraceptive effectiveness. *Contraceptive effectiveness* is defined as the proportion (or percentage) by which natural fecundability is reduced as a result of contraception. If effectiveness is $e\%$, then the natural fecundability f_n of the users is lowered to $f_n(1 - e/100)$ for all birth orders after the desired number of births has been reached.

Induced abortion is used exclusively by a certain proportion of the contraceptors. All conceptions after a given number of unwanted births are aborted. An additional input parameter defines this number. Some of these intended interruptions of pregnancy are obviated by spontaneous abortions occurring in the first 2 months of pregnancy. All pregnancies surviving into the third month are terminated by an induced abortion in that month, followed by 1 month of postabortion anovulation and return to the fecundable state.

To exercise the birth control option, separate calculations of reproductive histories for each subgroup of women with a particular number of desired births are made and their weighted average is taken. The output of the complete simulation includes age-specific induced abortion rates, proportions using contraception by age, and rates of unwanted births. A limitation of the birth control option is that it does not provide for the deliberate spacing of desired births, a limitation removed in the elaborations to be described in Chapter 7.

AGE SPECIFICITY

Because the differential equations of the reproductive process allow variation over age in the input parameters, two age functions have been included for greater realism:

1. *Natural fecundability*. In near conformity with a pattern suggested by Henry (1965), natural fecundability is assumed 0 before age 12, increasing linearly from 12 to 20, remaining constant at its "plateau value" from 20 to

30, and declining linearly to 0 at age 48. The plateau level between ages 20 and 30 is an input parameter specified before the simulation starts.

2. *Risk of spontaneous abortion.* The age-specific probability that a pregnancy is terminated by a spontaneous abortion is calculated from the J-shaped curve proposed by Nortman (1974) with a mean (over ages 20–40 years) determined by an input parameter.[5]

An earlier version of REPMOD carried a third age function designed to render age-dependent the mean length of the postpartum infecundable period. Reasons have been given in Chaper 2 for believing that postpartum anovulation is less sensitive to age than was originally thought.

MARITAL DISRUPTION

All married women in every reproductive state are subjected to the risk of becoming a widow or a divorcee. The risk of becoming a widow (by age) is taken from a model male lifetable where males are a predetermined number of years older than their spouses. For women who remarry, the time lost between marriages is assumed negligible. The risk of remarriage as well as the risks of marital disruption are permitted to vary with age. Output includes the proportions of cohort members in various marital statuses by year of life.

VALIDATION OF THE MODEL

In a 1977 paper, Bongaarts described the original version of REPMOD and simultaneously presented the first detailed fitting of a set of fertility observations on the basis of a macrosimulation model most of whose components are estimated indirectly from a variety of sources. For purposes of this fitting, he chose from a larger sample of eighteenth-century Canadian geneological records those 512 first marriages ostensibly having complete information and enduring until the wife reached age 45, thereby removing widowhood, divorce, and remarriage as complicating factors. Actual ages at marriage were utilized rather than predictions from a fitted Coale–McNeil first marriage curve. A mean fecundability of .31 was derived from analysis of the first birth intervals, this mean being well above most empirical esti-

---

[5] Let a denote the average risk of intrauterine mortality over ages 20–40. Then according to Nortman's function, that risk in the xth year of life is given by

$$a(x) = (0.805 + .004(x - 21.4)^2) .84 a.$$

This age-specific risk is minimal at ages 21 and 22. For example, if a = .17, which will be used as a standard input, $a(22)$ = .11. As age advances into the thirties and forties, $a(x)$ increases rapidly. To take the extreme, $a(50)$ = .58. Correspondingly, as age declines from 21 to 12 years, $a(x)$ progressively rises from .11 to .17.

mates. With other fecundity components put into what was then considered standard form, the last step of his fitting procedure consisted of determining iteratively that mean value (9.6 months) of postpartum anovulation that, together with all the other estimates, yielded the observed mean final parity of 6.46.

Though a match between model prediction and observation was guaranteed with respect to average completed family size, it is impressive that good agreement extended to such diverse aspects as age and age-parity-specific birth rates, final parity distribution, and duration-specific birth rates within 5-years age-of-marriage cohorts.

An especially encouraging implication is the essential soundness, under conditions of natural fertility, of assuming that the four main reproductive components operate independently of each other, excepting the dependence of gestational and anovulatory lengths on outcome of pregnancy.

That the validation test of REPMOD demonstrated a near approach to independence among risk of intrauterine mortality, length of postpartum anovulation, and natural fecundability when wife's age is held constant is not so startling when one considers their primary determinants: genetic defects of the embryo, breastfeeding practices, and coital frequency, respectively. Clearly these sets of forces could operate with a considerable degree of randomness relative to each other.

Nevertheless, such simplicity does not strictly exist in real life. Anderson (1975) has shown that natural fertility rates depend also on husband's age though not nearly so closely as wife's age. Under natural fertility conditions, last birth intervals tend to be longer than would be expected on age considerations alone, and, to a lesser extent, this is true of penultimate birth intervals. To explain this behavior, Leridon (1977, Appendix A) found it necessary to postulate that fecundity is sensitive to the approach of onset of natural sterility as well as to wife's age. It would seem that some sterilizing conditions are progressive with the last birth interval most seriously affected. Page (1977) has documented with Swedish data a secondary dependence of natural fertility on marriage duration. Further evidence is cited by Menken (1979). One suspects that coital frequency, the primary determinant of natural fecundability, might be responsive to interval from marriage as well as to ages of the spouses.

In its simulation of natural fertility, REPMOD treats like aged couples as heterogeneous with respect to natural fecundability. James (1961) and Leridon (1976) have produced evidence that couples vary in their risks of intrauterine mortality as well. It may be further suspected that women differ systematically in breastfeeding behavior and in their amenorrheic response to lactation, but there are not yet the prospective data spanning two consecutive, untruncated birth intervals to settle this issue. However, as remarked by Jacquard and Leridon (1973), the substantial .41 coefficient of variation estimated for natural fecundability may constitute the surrogate for the joint expression of all sources of persistent heterogeneity.

Differences between the version of REPMOD designed to fit the eighteenth-century Canadian sample and the standard version described earlier in this chapter and to be employed in the next section are four in number. First, a slightly different schedule of age at onset of natural sterility, taken from Henry (1965) instead of from Henry (1961), is to be used, but the changes here are trivial. Second, being exchanged for the very high mean plateau fecundability of .31 is that value, which, together with other assumptions, yields a TF of 15.3 births, an estimate to be derived in the next section of this chapter. At the same time the span of plateau fecundability is contracted from 15 years, ages 20–35, to the 10 years between 20 and 30 years. Third, for reasons given in Chapter 2, the mean risk of intrauterine mortality (for ages 20–40) is dropped from .24 to .17. Fourth, the age function of postpartum anovulation is made constant rather than linearly rising.

APPLICATION TO FECUNDITY

Fecundity, interpreted as natural fertility freed from the inhibitions of either delayed or broken marriages or lactational amenorrhea, is a theoretical concept for which there are no empirical observations. However, fecundity may be simulated by REPMOD and there is interest in doing so to see how wide is the associated spread of completed family sizes.

For this purpose, use of contraception, induced abortion, and sterilization is made 0. Divorce and widowhood are also banished. Postpartum anovulation is set at an average length of 1.5 months to reflect the absence of breastfeeding. The standard age functions described earlier, pertaining to risk of spontaneous pregnancy wastage and onset of natural sterility, are posited. Three equally weighted natural fecundability cohorts, having plateau values of $0.5f_n$, f_n, and $1.5f_n$, are distinguished, their respective natural fecundabilities following the standard age curve have been described. Consistent with a calculation in Chapter 4, age at marriage is set at 15 years for all women. This convention yields a fertility rate for age class 15–19 that is close to three-quarters of the fertility rate for age class 20–24.

As a final step in the operationalization of fecundity by means of REPMOD, the average plateau value f of natural fecundability is determined as that probability taken to two decimal places that in combination with all the other assumptions yields a TF closest to 15.3. This value turns out to be .19.[6]

[6] Sensitivity of TF to the value assigned to mean plateau fecundability f is as follows:

f	TF	ΔTF	f	TF	ΔTF
.17	14.50		.20	15.55	.33
.18	14.87	.37	.21	15.87	.32
.19	15.22	.35	.22	16.17	.30

Table 6.1

FREQUENCY DISTRIBUTIONS OF CHILDREN EVER BORN, UNDER FECUNDITY
CONDITIONS, BY SOURCE OF VARIATION ELIMINATED

Number of births	None of three sources eliminated	Source R.L. [a] eliminated	Source H.F. [b] eliminated	Sources R.L. and H.F. eliminated
0	20		20	
1	1		1	
2	3		3	
3	6		5	
4	6		5	
5	7		6	
6	10	2	7	
7	14	6	8	
8	20	16	10	
9	31	34	13	1
10	44	54	18	4
11	57	68	26	16
12	65	71	41	47
13	67	67	63	107
14	65	71	91	182
15	65	88	122	229
16	69	110	144	208
17	75	124	145	132
18	79	123	120	56
19	78	97	81	15
20	72	51	43	2
21	60	15	18	
22	43	2	6	
23	26		2	
24	12			
25	4			
26	1			
Total	1000	999	998	999

[a] R.L. signifies reproductive length.

[b] H.F. denotes heterogeneity of fecundability.

The associated frequency distribution of final parties is given in the first
column of Table 6.1 and several summary coefficients in the first column of
Table 6.2. Exhibiting an awesome range of 0–26 births, the distribution of
completed family sizes has a standard deviation of 5.09. By virtue of negative skewness, its mode of 18 births stands well above the median of 15.8 and
mean of 15.2. An interquartile range of 7.1 births is necessary to encompass
the central 50% of family sizes.

One might have expected a much tighter clustering of final parities around
the mean of 15.2. Accordingly, it is worth investigating the basis of such an
extreme variation in number of children ever born. Three components are
advantageously distinguished. First is variability of reproductive length.
This variation is being underestimated by the assumption of a constant age at
start of reproductive capacity, but the underestimate is not serious, being

Table 6.2

SUMMARY COEFFICIENTS OF DISTRIBUTIONS OF CHILDREN EVER BORN,
UNDER FECUNDITY CONDITIONS, BY SOURCE OF VARIATION ELIMINATED

Coefficient	None of three sources eliminated	Source R.L. [c] eliminated	Source H.F. [d] eliminated	Sources R.L. and H.F. eliminated
Mean	15.22	15.13	15.15	15.09
Mode	18.00	17.00	17.00	15.00
Standard deviation	5.09	3.35	4.02	1.73
Coefficient of variation	.33	.22	.27	.11
Skewness [a]	-.67	-.40	-1.63	-.16
Range	26.00	16.00	23.00	11.00
Q_3-Q_1 [b]	7.1	5.3	4.0	2.3

[a] $\Sigma(X-\bar{X})^3/\sigma^3 n$

[b] Interquartile range encompassing central 50%.

[c] R.L. signifies reproductive length.

[d] H.F. signifies heterogeneity of fecundability.

almost certainly less than 10%.[7] Second is hterogeneity with respect to natural fecundability, expressed as three cohorts having plateau fecundabilities standing in a relationship of 0.5, 1.0, and 1.5 to each other, over all ages. A third and residual source comprises the variability of conceptive delays and differing amounts of pregnancy wastage experienced within each fecundability cohort. While the first two sources relate to systematic differences among couples, the third source represents the operation of chance factors.

To assess the role of variable reproductive length, we compare the final parity distributions when reproductive length is allowed to vary and when it is fixed at that value in months that yields a total fecundity rate closest to 15.3. Meeting this requirement is a reproductive period that starts at 15 years of age and ends at 40, giving a length of 25 years. The comparison is given in Columns 1 and 2 of Tables 6.1 and 6.2. The standard deviation is reduced 34% from 5.09 to 3.35, and the coefficient of variation correspondingly from .33 to .22. The most striking effect is the reduction of range from 26 to 16 births by virtue of eliminating the smallest family sizes, namely all families having less than 5 children, as well as the largest families of 23 births or more. The degree of negative skewness is slightly reduced. The interquartile range slips from 7.1 births to 5.3.

[7] Suppose that start of reproductive capacity is abrupt, is uniformly distributed among women between ages 12 and 20 years, and is independent of ages at onset of natural sterility. Though almost certainly exaggerated, the variance of these starting ages, $8^2/12 = 5.33$, proves nevertheless to be well under 10% of the variance contributed by ages at onset of natural sterility.

Next we compare final parity distributions when fecundability is heterogeneous (characterized by plateau values of .095, .190, and .285 weighted equally) and when it is homogeneous (single plateau value of .17). By comparing Columns 1 and 3 of Tables 6.1 and 6.2, it is seen that the standard deviation is reduced from 5.09 to 4.02, or about 20%, an appreciable amount, but the reduction in range of family sizes is only from 26 to 23. Negative skewness is enhanced. Eliminating the high fecundability cohort attenuates the right tail of very large families whereas the presence of variable reproductive length essentially preserves the left tail of small families.

The significance of chance factors is evaluated by comparing the values of Columns 1 of Tables 6.1 and 6.2 with those of Columns 4, generated when fecundability is made homogeneous (with a plateau value of .17) and the limits of the reproductive period are fixed at 15 and 40 years of age. The removal of systematic differences among couples reduces the standard deviation of children ever born by two-thirds from 5.09 to 1.73. Negative skewness is largely eliminated. The range retreats from 26 to 11. Family size now ranges from 9 to 20 births.

Though greatly diminished, this residual variability, attributable entirely to chance factors, remains impressive. Why is the effect of chance factors so large? Under fecundity conditions, the variability of intervals from marriage to first birth or from first to second birth are fairly modest, respective standard deviations having an order of magnitude around 6 months. However, given a homogeneous population of couples, the lengths of two consecutive birth intervals will be uncorrelated, and as a result the two intervals added together will have a variance that is the sum of the variances of the individual intervals. More generally, among these homogeneous couples the time required for n births in an unlimited reproductive period will have a variance n times that of a single birth interval. That is, chance variation accumulates over multiple births, and the opportunities for such cumulation are substantial when the average number of births is as high as 15. More to the point, the chance variation governs how many births can be fitted into a 25-year reproductive period.

To summarize our findings about fertility under the hypothetical conditions of fecundity, not only is the mean number of births at 15.2 very large, but the scatter around it is commensurately large, featuring a range of 0–26 children ever born. Systematic factors account for about two-thirds of the variability; chance factors, one-third. Of the two sources of systematic variation, variability of reproductive length plays the dominant role and heterogeneity of fecundability an important secondary role.

NATURAL FERTILITY

Compared with fecundity, natural fertility involves two additional variables: (a) varying age of first marriages as well as interregnums of nonmarriage dependent on divorce, widowhood, and remarriage; and (*b*) prolonging of postpartum anovulation by lactation. To simplify discussion, let us exclude divorce and widowhood (and hence the opportunity for remarriage).

The two new components of variation both act to reduce total fertility. Any delaying of first marriage foreshortens the reproductive period. Longer postpartum anovulation lengthens individual birth intervals.

The net effect of the two added factors on variation of final family size is less easily predicted. Variable age of marriage tends to augment the variability of the reproductive period. The dispersion of individual birth intervals is enhanced by the differing durations of postpartum anovulation. However, there is now a lower average number of birth intervals over which to cumulate the chance variation of individual intervals.

Fortunately natural fertility is accessible to empirical study. An interesting population because of extremely long postpartum anovulation and low natural fecundability is that of Bangladesh. This population, which at least in its rural majority continues to approximate natural fertility conditions, commands demographic importance because of its large size. It will be of interest in Chapters 7 and 8 to contrast what will be called the "peasant" context (illustrated by Bangladesh and representing relatively low natural fertility on account of lengthy amenorrhea and low natural fecundability) with the "modern" or industrial context (illustrated by the United States and featuring a somewhat higher natural fecundability [mean plateau value of .19 instead of .16] and a mean length of postpartum anovulation of only 3.0 months, reflective of mostly brief or absent lactation).

In the present section, the details of fitting the Bangladesh population are given and the sources of the large variation in completed family size are then explored.

Principal reliance is placed on the results of the 1975 Bangladesh *World Fertility Survey* (hereafter abbreviated as WFS). For wives currently married and aged 40–44 years, mean final parity is 7.6. Wives 45 years and over report a somewhat smaller number of children ever born, 7.3, which strongly suggests underreporting. Hence it will be the fertility of the former group that is fitted.

The retrospective data gathered in the WFS on marriage age are considered not entirely reliable, and the best estimates would seem to be ones derived from census data. Singulate mean age of marriage is estimated at 13 years for 1931, 14 years from three estimates spanning the period 1941–1961, and 15 up to 16 years in the period 1965–1975 (Miranda, 1980). During 1945–1950 when the bulk of the cohort of wives aged 40–44 in 1975 were marrying, the mean age of marriage was apparently slightly over 14 years. As there is quite often a delay between the formal marriage ceremony and consummation, and as some brides may not have reached menarche, it seems not unreasonable to set the input parameter $\bar{a}$ for mean age of marriage at a slightly higher age, namely 16 years. The parameter a_0, denoting earliest age of marriage, properly receives a low value, such as 11. Given the near universality of marriage, parameter C for the proportion ultimately marrying is set at 1.0. Based on WFS breastfeeding data, Bongaarts and Kirmeyer (1982) estimate mean postpartum anovulation at 18.64. This value is rounded to 18.5 in REPMOD.[8]

As a final step, with other factors taken in their standard patterns, including the age schedule of onset of natural sterility, level and age pattern or risk of spontaneous intrauterine mortality, heterogeneous level ($.5f_n$, f_n, and $1.5f_n$) and age pattern of natural fecundability, and conditional lengths of gestation and postpartum anovulation (and with contraception, induced abortion, widowhood, and divorce all banished), it is found that the mean plateau fecundability (taken to two decimal places) best fitting the observed TFR of 7.6 is .16. That this estimate is somewhat below the value of .19 estimated from the investigation of the TF, in the previous section, is most readily explained by the phenomenon of seasonal separation of spouses that has been demonstrated in the Matlab area (Chen, Ahmed, Gesche, and Mosely 1974) and may well characterize broad segments of the rural Bangladesh population.

The simulated and empirical distributions of final parity are juxtaposed in Table 6.3. Total fertility rates are both 7.6. The empirical distribution exhibits a barely larger variability than its simulated counterpart and has a mode of 9 children rather than 8. On the whole, the correspondence is quite close.

An additional check on the appropriateness of the three marriage parameters a_0, $\bar{a}$, and C chosen is the parity distribution of wives reporting ages under 15. Seventy-seven out of 1000 have already reached parity one. The simulated counterpart is 73, indicating extremely good agreement. It was found that employing a_0 values higher than 11 yielded underestimates of this early fertility, and, even more significantly, by rendering marriage age less variable, relative to its mean, these higher a_0 values generated too small a scatter of completed family sizes.

The simulated distribution of children ever born is repeated in Column 1 of Table 6.4 and the associated summary coefficients are given in the corresponding column of Table 6.5. Lengthy postpartum anovulation offsetting early and universal marriage with no marital disruption until age 50 generates a moderately high TFR of 7.59 births. Primarily because of the very long

---

[8] The function being used in REPMOD to simulate distributions of postpartum anovulation tends to exaggerate variability when the mean is appreciably longer than 14 months (Potter and Kobrin 1981). However this exaggeration applies only to distributions of amenorrhea freed of the effects of infant mortality. Plainly, the WFS distribution of final parities being fitted is very much affected by infant mortality and indeed, very high infant mortality. In the presence of such high infant mortality, the variance of postpartum anovulation can be expected to increase substantially owing to the superimposition of a second mode at Months 1 and 2, remote from the principal mode in the vicinity of Months 18 and 19. That the variance of postpartum anovulation is not being seriously inflated is suggested by the fact that in Table 6.3 the simulated distribution of final parity has a slightly smaller variance than the WFS distribution.

Table 6.3

SURVEYED AND SIMULATED DISTRIBUTIONS OF CHILDREN EVER BORN AMONG CURRENTLY MARRIED BANGLADESH WOMEN, AGED 40–44 YEARS[a]

Children ever born	Observed WFS distribution	Simulated by REPMOD
0	23	23
1	12	8
2	19	14
3	39	22
4	29	40
5	63	74
6	115	117
7	144	152
8	158	164
9	173	152
10	95	117
11 or more	130	116
Total	1000	999

[a] World Fertility Survey, "Bangladesh Fertility Survey 1975, First Report," Ministry of Health and Population Control, Government of the People's Republic of Bangladesh, December, 1978.

Table 6.4

FREQUENCY DISTRIBUTIONS OF CHILDREN EVER BORN, UNDER NATURAL FERTILITY CONDITIONS, BY SOURCE OF VARIATION ELIMINATED

Number of births	None of three sources eliminated	Source R.L. [a] eliminated	Source H.F. [a] eliminated	Source R.L. and H.F. eliminated
0	23		23	
1	8		7	
2	14		13	
3	22	3	19	
4	40	20	31	3
5	74	72	57	33
6	117	154	104	145
7	152	229	166	303
8	164	250	206	311
9	152	179	187	159
10	117	75	118	40
11	71	17	51	5
12	32	2	15	
13	11		3	
14	2			
15				
16				
17				
Total	999	1001	1000	999

[a] Initials R.L. and H.F. stand for reproductive length and heterogeneity of fecundability.

Table 6.5
SUMMARY COEFFICIENTS OF DISTRIBUTION OF CHILDREN EVER BORN
UNDER NATURAL FERTILITY CONDITIONS, BY SOURCE OF VARIATION
ELIMINATED

Coefficient	None of three sources eliminated	Source R.L. a/ eliminated	Source H.F. a/ eliminated	Source R.L. and H.F. eliminated
Mean	7.59	7.54	7.58	7.55
Mode	8.00	8.00	8.00	8.00
Standard deviation	2.61	1.53	2.37	1.19
Coefficient of variation	.34	.20	.31	.16
Skewness	−.59	−.10	−.96	.02
Range	14.00	9.00	2.70	1.63
$Q_3 - Q_1$	3.30	2.12	2.70	1.63

a/ Initials R.L. and H.F. signify reproductive length and heterogeneity
of fecundability.

anovulation and secondarily because of the slightly lower fecundability
levels, this TFR of 7.59 is only half the fecundity level of 15.20. Nevertheless
the range of final parity is impressive, extending from 0 to 14 births. The
standard deviation of 2.61 is appreciably below the 5.09 characterizing
fecundity conditions. Thus the additional contributions to variability by increased postpartum anovulation and variable marriage age are more than
compensated for by the reduced number of births over which chance variation is being accumulated. Interestingly though, comparisons of Columns 1
of Table 6.2 and 6.5 show virtually equal coefficients of variation and of
negative skewness under fecundity and natural fertility conditions.

Once more it is of interest to partition total variability of children never
born into three components. The four columns of Table 6.4 and 6.5 afford
parallel comparisons to those of Tables 6.1 and 6.2. This time reproductive
length is rendered more variable by differing ages of marriage. The definition
of heterogeneity of fecundability remains unchanged. The component of
residual chance variation is augmented by appreciably varying postpartum
anovulation.

In order to generate TFRs as close to 7.59 as possible, reproductive length
in Columns 2 and 4 of Tables 6.4 and 6.5 is assigned limits of 16 and 40 years,
whereas in Columns 3 and 4, homogeneous fecundability is represented by a
plateau value of .14.

To a considerable extent the differentials according to which sources of
variability are eliminated are the same for fecundity and natural fertility.
Chance factors account for about 45% of the total standard deviation in the

simulated Bangladesh population, somewhat more than the 33% they account for under fecundity conditions. Once again, reproductive length constitutes a more important source of systematic variation than heterogeneous fecundability. More particularly, the variability of reproductive length largely accounts for the negative skewness of the distribution of children ever born. The highest degree of negative skewness is found when heterogeneous fecundability alone is eliminated as a source of variability. Chance factors operating by themselves generate an imposing range of 4–11 children.

SUMMARY

This and the succeeding three chapters carry two main interests that contrast with the emphasis placed on aggregate fertility of the five preceding chapters. First is a focus on fertility variation among individual couples of a population; second is a consideration of the conditions necessary for specified degrees of fertility control, the areas of control being family size, birth spacing, and sex preselection.

Three kinds of reproductive models—all capable of encompassing systematic as well as stochastic elements—namely, analytical models, macrosimulation, and Monte Carlo microsimulation—are distinguished. Reasons for relying so heavily on a particular macrosimulation model, REPMOD, are cited. The simplest and the standard versions of REPMOD are described in detail. However, even the standard version proves imperfectly suited for most applications, and a series of adjustments of REPMOD, each tailored to a special purpose, have proven necessary and are delineated, mostly in footnotes, throughout Chapters 6–8.

REPMOD is first applied to fecundity, operationalized as natural fertility freed of the inhibitions of delayed or interrupted marriage and of lactational amenorrhea. The spread of family sizes proves awesome. When the sources of this variation are explored, it is found that systematic factors account for about two-thirds of the variability and chance factors one-third. Of the two sources of systematic variation, variability of reproductive length plays the dominant role and heterogeneity of natural fecundability an important secondary role.

Natural fertility, illustrated by a macrosimulation of the Bangladesh population, is analyzed in an analogous way. The mean level of natural fertility is only half that of fecundity because birth intervals are lengthened by prolonged postpartum anovulation and reproductive periods shortened by time spent outside of marriage. Nevertheless, the variation in number of births among couples remains imposing. In this case chance factors account for about 45% of the total standard deviation, and again, reproductive length constitutes a more important source of systematic variation than heterogeneous fecundability.

REFERENCES

Anderson, B. A. (1975), "Male Age and Fertility, Results from Ireland Prior to 1911," *Population Index, 41,* 4, 561–566.

Barrett, J. C. (1969), "A Monte Carlo Simulation of Human Reproduction," *Genus, 25,* 1–22.

Bodmer, W. F. and A. Jacquard (1968), "La Variance de la Dimension des Familles Selon Divers Facteurs de la Fecondite," *Population, 24* (Sept.–Oct.), 869–878.

Bongaarts, J. (1975), "A Method for the Estimation of Fecundability," *Demography, 12* (November), 645–660.

Bongaarts, J. (1977), "A Dynamic Model of the Reproductive Process," *Population Studies, 31* (March), 59–73.

Bongaarts, J. (1980), "The Fertility Inhibiting Effects of the Intermediate Fertility Variables," unpublished paper prepared for the IUSSP and WFS Seminar on the Analysis of Maternity Histories, London, April.

Bongaarts, J. and S. W. Kirmeyer (1982), "Estimating the Impact of Contraceptive Prevalence on Fertility: Aggregate and Age Specific Versions of a Model," in *The Role of Surveys in the Analysis of Family Planning Programs,* A. Hermalin and B. Entwisle, Eds. Ordina Liege.

Chen, L. C., S. Ahmed, M. Gesche, and W. H. Mosely (1974), "A Prospective Study of Birth Interval Dynamics in Rural Bangladesh," *Population Studies, 28* (July), 277–298.

Coale, A. J. (1971), "Age Patterns of Marriage," *Population Studies, 25,* 2 (July), 193–214.

Coale, A. J. (1977), "The Development of New Models of Nuptiality and Fertility," *Population, 32,* Numero Special, (September), 131–154.

Coale, A. J. and D. R. McNeil (1972), "The Distribution by Age of the Frequency of First Marriage in a Female Cohort," *Journal of the American Statistical Association, 67,* 743–749.

Ford, K. (1976), "Abortion and Family Building Models: Fertility Limitation in Hungary," *Demography, 13* (Nov.), 495–506.

Henry, L. (1961), "Some Data on Natural Fertility," *Eugenics Quarterly, 8* (June), 81–91.

Henry, L. (1965), "French Statistical Research in Natural Fertility," in M. C. Sheps and J. C. Ridley, eds., *Public Health and Population Change,* University of Pittsburgh Press, Pittsburgh, pp. 333–350.

Holmberg, I. (1972), "Fecundity, Fertility and Family Planning. Applications of Demographic Micro-models," Vols. I (1970) and II (1972), Demographic Institute, University of Gottenburg, Sweden.

Jacquard, M. A. (1967), "La Reproduction Humaine en Regime Malthusian," *Population, 22* (Sept.–Oct.) 5, 897–920.

Jacquard, A. and H. Leridon (1973), "Simulating Human Reproduction: How Complicated Should a Model Be?" in B. Dyke and J. W. MacCluer, Eds., *Computer Simulation in Human Population Studies,* Academic Press, New York, pp. 241–249.

James, W. H. (1961), "On the Possibility of Segregation in the Propensity to Spontaneous Abortion in the Human Female," *Annals of Human Genetics, 25,* 207–213.

Lachenbruch, P. A., M. C. Sheps, and A. M. Sorant (1973), "Applications of POPREP, A Modification of POPSIM," in B. Dyke and J. W. MacCluer, Eds., *Computer Simulation in Human Population Studies,* Academic Press, Inc., New York, pp. 305–328.

Leridon, H. (1976), "Facts and Artifacts in the Study of Intrauterine Mortality: A Reconsideration of Pregnancy Histories." *Population Studies, 30* (July), pp. 319–336.

Leridon, H. (1977), *Human Fertility: The Basic Components*, University of Chicago Press, Chicago and London.

Menken, J. (1979), "Introduction," in H. Leridon and J. Menken, eds., *Natural Fertility*, Ordina Editions, Liege Belgium, pp. 3–13.

Miranda, A. (1980), "Nuptiality in Bangladesh," *The Journal of Social Studies, 9* (July), 58–98.

Nortman, D. (1974), "Parental Age as a Factor in Pregnancy Outcome and Child Development," *Reports on Population/Family Planning, 16* (August).

Page, H. J. (1977), "Patterns Underlying Fertility Schedules: A Decomposition by Age and Marriage Duration," *Population Studies, 31* (March), 85–106.

Potter, R. G. (1969), "Renewal Theory and Births Averted," *International Population Conference: London, 1969*, International Union for the Scientific Study of the Population, Liege, Vol. 1, pp. 145–150.

Potter, R. G. (1971), "Inadequacy of an One-Method Family Planning Program," *Studies in Family Planning, 2* (January), 1–5.

Potter, R. G. (1972), "Additional Births Averted When Abortion Is Added to Contraception," *Studies in Family Planning, 3* (April), 53–59.

Potter, R. G. and F. E. Kobrin (1981), "Distributions of Amenorrhea and Anovulation," *Population Studies, 35,* (March), 85–99.

Potter, R. G. and M. P. Parker (1964), "Predicting the Time Required to Conceive," *Population Studies, 18* (July), 99–116.

Potter, R. G. and J. M. Sakoda (1966), "A Computer Model of Family Building Based on Expected Values," *Demography, 3,* 2, 450–461.

Potter, R. G. and J. M. Sakoda (1967), "Family Planning and Fecundity," *Population Studies, 20* (March), 311–328.

Potter, R. G., J. M. Sakoda, and W. E. Feinberg (1968), "Variable Fecundability and the Timing of Births," *Eugenics Quarterly, 15* (September), 155–163.

Ridley, J. C. and M. C. Sheps (1966), "An Analytic Simulation Model of Human Reproduction with Demographic and Biological Components," *Population Studies, 19* (March), 297–310.

Sheps, M. C. (1964), "On the Time Required for Conception," *Population Studies, 18* (July), 85–97.

Sheps, M. C. and Jane A. Menken (1973). *Mathematical Models of Conception and Birth*, University of Chicago Press, Chicago.

Smith, T. E. (1966), "The Cocos-Keeling Islands: A Demographic Laboratory," *Population Studies, 14* (November), 94–130.

Tuan, C. H. (1958), "Reproductive Histories of Chinese Women in Rural Taiwan," *Population Studies, 12* (July), 40–50.

VanGinneken, J. K. (1978), "The Impact of Prolonged Breast Feeding on Birth Interval and on Postpartum Amenorrhea," in W. H. Mosley, Ed, *Nutrition and Human Reproduction*, New York, Plenum, pp. 179–196.

Venkatacharya, K. (1971), "Fertility and Fecundability," *Social Biology, 18,* 406–415.

World Fertility Survey (1978), *Bangladesh Fertility Survey, 1975: First Report*, Ministry of Health and Population Control, Government of the People's Republic of Bangladesh, December.

7
Family-Size Control

INTRODUCTION

Control by a married couple of their family size has two aspects: attaining the number of children they want and then avoiding additional unwanted births. The results of Chapter 6 make clear that unless a large family is aspired to, a far higher proportion of couples will face the problem of avoiding excess fertility than will be frustrated by an incapacity to have all the children they want.

In the analyses of this chapter, no account will be taken of the family-size ambiguities consequent upon a child's death or changes of mind with respect to, or spouse disagreement concerning, number of children wanted. It will be assumed that the couple agree on their family-size objective, which remains constant during a marriage that survives intact until the end of the reproductive period.

Given these simplified conditions, then, with other factors constant, the fraction of couples thwarted for physiological reasons from having all the children they want is higher with (a) later marriage; (b) longer deferral of childbearing in marriage; (c) more children wanted; (d) wider spacing sought between desired births; or (e) more efficient contraception practiced in behalf of the spacing goal. Nevertheless, it will be demonstrated that unless the first three factors conspire to extend childbearing into the last third of the reproductive period, the couple can afford to space desired births 2 or 3 years without appreciably increasing risks of not attaining intended family size. It turns out that the few years added by deliberately spacing births usually still allows the mother to have her last desired birth at an age when natural sterility risks are low.

The causal mechanism underlying subfertility is an onset of natural sterility earlier than the potential age of attaining desired family size. Although most couples do not lose reproductive capacity until the wife is in her late thirties or early forties (see Chapter 2), a minority have this happen earlier. Any combination of factors making for a later expected age at last-desired child can only raise the proportion subfertile.

Two additional factors contributing to a later potential age at end of desired childbearing is lower than average natural fecundability, which tends to contribute longer conceptive delays when contraception is waived or else deliberately interrupted, and adverse luck in the shape of longer conceptive delays or more spontaneous pregnancy losses than would be expected from the couple's fecundity. The reproductive model REPMOD permits one to calculate what might have been the mean age at attainment of desired family size of those suffering subfertility as well as the corresponding mean for those who succeed in reaching their family-size goal. If it can be shown that in a cohort of couples made homogeneous with respect to such factors as marriage age, family size, and spacing goals, and effectiveness of contraception, these two average ages are only trivially apart, then one has demonstrated that the two factors of luck and variation in natural fecundability are secondary whereas the predominant determinant of subfertility is earliness of onset of natural sterility.

With a shift of context from the United States to Bangladesh, it will be shown that seeking n boys (or n girls) occasions more subfertility than seeking $2n$ children without regard to sex composition. The reason is the highly variable number of children needed to realize the nth child of the designated sex. For the unlucky minority who require well over $2n$ children to achieve their objective, the risk of subfertility becomes substantial. In this manner a sex compositional goal weakens family-size control.

When simulating excess fertility, it has proven expedient to treat the incidence of unwanted births as a function of three sets of factors: (a) length of risk period (i.e., intervals from attainment of desired family size to onset of natural sterility) and fecundity during it; (b) effectiveness of contraception (including possibly sterilization and induced abortion); and (c) chance factors. The macrosimulation REPMOD makes it possible to vary the first two sets of systematic factors from cohort to cohort and to gauge their impact by examining the resultant variation in mean excess births per capita among couples attaining desired family size. The role of chance factors may be assessed by inspecting the dispersion of excess births among couples belonging to a homogeneous cohort. Fortunately, factors such as marriage age, spacing, and family-size goals, and effectiveness of contraception practiced for spacing purposes do not have to be varied individually since their joint relevance can be operationalized as wife's age at start of risk period.

A central point demonstrated is that even when the effectiveness of contraception is high, and therefore the monthly risk of an unintended conception low, because the typical risk period encompasses so many months of exposure, the probability of one or more contraceptive failures can be quite high. This dolorous axiom of fertility control is not new. It was rehearsed 15 years ago (Potter and Sakoda, 1966 and 1967) but on the basis of a model of reproduction less realistic than REPMOD.

This chapter, perhaps the most difficult in the book, is organized in the following manner. Modifications of the standard version of REPMOD are necessary in order to incorporate spacing as well as family-size goals into its simulation. These elaborations are broadly defined in the next section, although most of the details are dealt with by a series of footnotes. Subfertility aspects are next examined, first in the U.S. context with primacy given to the role of early sterility and then secondly in the Bangladesh context, the augmenting of subfertility by sex compositional goals being illustrated.

The treatment of excess fertility, which takes up the larger half of the chapter, is organized into four sections. Matters relating to the risk period and potential fertility during it are addressed first. Available in the literature for the United States are lifetable cumulative pregnancy rates while practicing designated contraceptives. For use as input in REPMOD, these curves have to be converted into estimates of average contraceptive effectiveness. This conversion is considered in a relatively technical section titled "contraceptive effectiveness." In the same section, three standards of protection against unwanted births, namely means of .20, .38, and .50 excess births per couple attaining desired family size, are derived from the reports of U.S. respondents concerning their family limitation during the 1970s.

It is shown, in the following section, that at the average effectiveness reported in the literature, nonpermanent contraception alone does not suffice to meet the lowest of the three standards of protection. Repeated abortion alone is an even less plausible instrumentality on account of the appalling number of operations per couple that would be called for. Only when one adds in sterilization at the incidences reported as well as an abortion accompaniment is a reasonable fit obtained between the standards of family limitation claimed by respondents and those generated by REPMOD simulations.

The last section deals briefly with three supplementary points having to do with the timing of excess births, the extra unwanted births associated with marriages precipitated by premarital pregnancy, and in the Bangladesh context, the significance of lengthy postpartum anovulation for lowering excess fertility.

This relatively long and difficult chapter ends with a summary to which the general reader might want to turn next.

OPERATIONALIZATION

The standard version of REPMOD enables one to simulate contraception or abortion practiced to limit births once the parity equivalent to desired family size is reached. By this approach, Tietze and Bongaarts (1975) have explored the requirements for replacement-level fertility. They distinguished three family-planning strategies: contraception alone; repeated induced abortion alone; and contraception backed by induced abortion. The authors demonstrate that, at empirically estimated levels of effectiveness, a strategy of exclusive reliance on contraception proves inadequate in the sense that the majority of couples will sustain heavy excess fertility. An exclusive reliance on induced abortion is even less satisfactory because as a vehicle of replacement-level fertility it calls for wholly implausible numbers of deliberate pregnancy interruptions. It is concluded that no population has kept fertility close to the replacement standard without relying on a combination of contraception and induced abortion, the former to keep the number of excess pregnancies per couple at modest levels and the latter to prevent their eventuation into excess parturition. An earlier demonstration of the unsatisfactory protection vouchsafed by an exclusive regimen of either repeated abortion or contraception at empirical levels of effectiveness and continuation was obtained by a more limited model, ACCOFERT, simulating the efforts at family limitation of a cohort attaining desired family size at a given age (Potter 1971, 1972).

Striking though the results of Tietze and Bongaarts be, it may be argued that they are slightly exaggerated by a failure to allow for birth-spacing efforts, which tend to shorten the risk period when excess fertility is a hazard. Then too, quite as important as the mean number of unwanted births per couple is the variation around this mean. A principal objective of the present chapter is to examine variation as well as mean values of excess fertility by means of an elaborated version of REPMOD encompassing spacing behavior.

To incorporate spacing behavior into REPMOD, appeal is made to what will be called the ''master schedule'' principle of spacing. This construct is discussed more thoroughly in Chapter 8 where it is contrasted with another spacing principle. The basic notion is that the couple have from marriage a time plan for their desired childbearing. Fixed in mind are preferred intervals between marriage and first birth and between consecutive desired births. If the couple fall behind schedule for reason of slow conception or spontaneous pregnancy wastage, they waive contraception until they catch up. If they get ahead by virtue of contraceptive failure, they try to prolong their next segment of contraception until 12 months short of the next targeted birth. As an example of a master schedule spacing goal, they might strive to have their first born 2 years after marriage and put 3 years between consecutive children. Alternatively they might elect not to delay the first child and have only 2 years between successive children.

It is well documented that couples spacing desired births practice less meticulous and therefore less effective contraception than couples trying to prevent unwanted children (Jones, Paul, and Westoff 1980, Sagi, Potter, and Westoff 1962). Accordingly, a distinction is made between "spacing effectiveness," denoted by "e_s," and "limiting effectiveness," denoted by "e_l," of contraception. By contraceptive effectiveness, of course, is meant the proportionate reduction of natural fecundability achieved by the practice of contraception, which, from Chapter 3, has the formula $e = 1 - f_r/f_n$. For example, if $f_n = .190$ and $f_r = .019$, $e = 1 - .019/.190 = .90$; that is, contraception is 90% effective for having reduced natural fecundability by 90%. In any run of REPMOD that simulates child spacing and family limitation, the two effectiveness parameters e_s and e_l may take different values as may the two parameters "MB" and "BB," standing respectively for preferred interval between marriage and first birth and preferred interval between consecutive births.

A price that has to be paid in any run of REPMOD simulating spacing behavior is to have a single age of marriage in order to establish a one-to-one relationship between current age of wife and marriage duration.[1] Apropos of master schedule spacing goals, it is further posited that if not ahead of their schedule, couples standardly interrupt contraception 1 year before the target date for their next birth, implying a confidence that they will conceive promptly once they seek a pregnancy.[2]

---

[1] It may be recalled from the description of the standard version of REPMOD in Chapter 6 that several fecundity parameters are age dependent and that the basic fertility results generated are jointly specified in terms of age and parity. To extend the specification to age, parity, *and* marriage duration would entail an enormous increase in program complexity and running expense. The most obvious way around this dilemma is to bring age and marriage duration into a one-to-one relationship, so that, from a knowledge of the wife's age, one immediately knows marriage duration and vice versa. The same kind of expensive elaboration would be necessary to achieve joint specificity with respect to age, parity (birth order), and pregnancy order, without which one cannot derive a distribution, but only a mean number of induced abortions. Unfortunately there appears to be no easy solution to this problem, and as a result when examining family planning strategies involving induced abortion, it is possible to derive only their mean number and not their distribution.

[2] Simulating spacing behavior is chiefly a matter of controlling at what durations the hypothetical couples are or are not practicing contraception. Recall that natural fecundability $f_n(a)$ varies with the wife's age a, and, therefore, residual fecundability $f_r(a) = (1 - e)f_n(a)$ is also age dependent. Assume a master-schedule spacing goal defined by parameters MB and BB, a desired family size of D births, and a marriage age M. Wife's current age a and parameters MB, BB, and M are all measured in months. Then so long as the couple's parity is 0, and marriage duration d (in months) is less than $MB - 12$ (which is to say that wife's age a is less than M + MB − 12), they practice contraception, that is, their fecundability is $f_r(a) = (1 - e_s)f_n(a)$. When $d > MB - 12$, natural fecundability $f_n(a)$ operates. Correspondingly, so long as their parity is k, $1 \leq k \leq D - 1$, and marriage duration is less than $MB + (k - 1)BB - 12$ (equivalent to $a \leq M + MB + (k - 1)BB - 12$), $f_r(a) = (1 - e_s)f_n(a)$ operates, but when the criterion duration is equalled or exceeded, natural fecundability $f_n(a)$ takes over again. For parities D or higher, when the couple are at the stage of seeking to avoid any further pregnancies, and therefore are operating under limiting effectiveness, residual fecundability, $f_r(a) = (1 - e_l)f_n(a)$, prevails.

SUBFERTILITY

The incidence of natural sterility by age of wife is most readily measured for populations practicing little or no birth control and not subject to sterilizing operations for medical or contraceptive reasons. Evidence of this type was reviewed in Chapter 2, suggesting that onset of natural sterility varies little among populations, except in cases where gonorrhea or genital tuberculosis are widespread. According to a careful estimate by Henry (1965), the incidence of natural sterility is about 3% when the wife is age 20, 5% when she is 25, and rises therafter to 8% at age 30, 15% at age 35, 32% at age 40, and, as a very rough order of magnitude, 69% at age 45, and virtually 100% by age 50. An age schedule of annual proportions sterile based on a curve drawn through the above seven proportions has been incorporated into REPMOD. Employed in Chapter 6, this age schedule will be used in the present and next chapter.[3]

The incidence of *subfertility,* an inability for physiological reasons to have all the children wanted, is difficult to measure in contemporary society. In nationally representative interview surveys, many respondents are in the early or middle stages of the reproductive period and for them apparent subfertility may or may not prove permanent. Even among respondents approaching menopausal age, allegations of not having all the children wanted may reflect feelings that they can not afford them economically, rather than representing physiological barriers that can not be corrected. Then too, sterilizing operations originally accepted in part for contraceptive reasons may later be rationalized as having had entirely a medical motivation.

Subfertility is not so much a matter of ''running out of time,'' that is, because of very low fecundity and not having reached desired family size at an advanced age when further childbearing is considered unacceptable, but rather reflects the more or less abrupt onset of natural sterility during the early or middle years of the reproductive span. This point is illustrated by the calculations of Chapter 6, which show that when reproductive length is fixed at 25 years, no family sizes smaller than three children are encountered under natural fertility conditions, and a minimum of six births is reached under fecundity conditions.

An older bridal age, more children sought, wider spacing preferred, and more effective contraception backing the spacing goal, all increase the proportion subfertile. For example, a woman who marries at 30 years and seeks

---

[3] Incidentally, regarding affluent societies, it is not at all clear that medical advances have succeeded in lowering the incidence of involuntary sterility in view of the large number of sterilizing operations for medical reasons. At least one condition frequently resulting in sterility, namely endometriosis, may be on the increase owing to the delaying of first pregnancies. Moreover, little or no medical progress has yet been made correcting male problems that are estimated to be the cause of couple sterility from one-third to one-half the time (McFalls 1979, Troen and Oshima 1980).

three widely spaced children, and therefore is ready not to complete her childbearing until her late thirties, runs a much higher risk of having her plans thwarted by sterility than the wife who wants two unspaced children to follow a marriage at age 20. The latter runs about a 3% risk of subfertility; the former a risk of nearly one-third. Chance factors may also play an adverse role when repeated pregnancy losses or slow conception put the couple behind their intended childbearing schedule. Of course, the risk of such adversity is enhanced by subfecundity in the form of either a special predisposition for pregnancy wastage or lower-than-average natural fecundability. Broadly, then, for any combination of family goals and marriage age, those who fail to attain desired family size are selected in varying degree for earlier-than-average onset of natural sterility, for subfecundity, and for ill luck in the shape of slower conception or more pregnancy wastage than is to be expected on the average from the couple's particular fecundity values.

The simulations based on REPMOD, which immediately follow, are designed to explore the sensitivity of subfertility to the factors of marriage age, intended family size, spacing goals, and effectiveness of contraception practiced for spacing purposes (spacing effectiveness). More particularly, does spacing desired births as opposed to having them as quickly as nature allows cause a significant rise in the proportion subject to subfertility?

Simulations for the United States

To represent a modern context, postpartum anovulation is set at a mean of 3.0 months, connoting absent or brief lactation. Otherwise the fecundity assumptions are those of the standard version of REPMOD defined earlier. Desired family size is taken as one, two, or three children. Encompassed by this range is the TFR of 1.8, estimated in Chapter 3 for U.S. couples in 1975. Three bridal ages at first marriage are considered: 20, 25, and 30 years. The first two bracket the singulate mean ages of first marriage of 20.5 and 22.4 years for U.S. couples in 1960 and 1977, respectively. Interpolated, these two estimates, cited in Chapter 3, indicate a mean age at first marriage of about 22.0 years for the early 1970s. *Narrow* spacing signifies no contraception practiced for spacing purposes, or equivalently, a spacing effectiveness of 0. A *medium*-spacing goal is defined as no interest in delaying the first born but a separation of 2 years sought between consecutive births. By a *wide*-spacing goal is meant that the couple seek to have their first child 2 years after marriage and to separate successive births by 3 years. The rationales behind these spacing goals are discussed in Chapter 8.

One might hypothesize that how much the risk of subfertility is raised by a wider spacing goal depends in part on spacing effectiveness. The theoretical limits of spacing effectiveness are 0 and 1.0. Taken as an intermediate, the estimate of spacing effectiveness is .90. Though this value may be regarded

Table 7.1
PROPORTION FAILING TO ATTAIN DESIRED FAMILY SIZE

Marriage age and number of children desired	No spacing	Medium spacing		Wide spacing	
		e = .90	e = 1.00	e = .90	e = 1.00
Marriage at age 20					
1 child desired	.030	.030	.030	.031	.031
2 children	.034	.037	.037	.045	.047
3 children	.043	.047	.048	.060	.062
Marriage at age 25					
1 child desired	.051	.051	.051	.055	.057
2 children	.061	.063	.063	.075	.078
3 children	.073	.081	.082	.108	.113
Marrage at age 30					
1 child desired	.088	.088	.088	.097	.099
2 children	.110	.115	.116	.146	.154
3 children	.147	.164	.167	.253	.269

as representative of U.S. couples in the 1960s, it is fairly certainly low for the early 1970s.[4] As will be seen, the proportions subfertile are relatively insensitive to this choice between .90 and 1.00.

In Table 7.1, based on a set of REPMOD runs, are given proportions of couples failing to reach desired family size as a function of marriage age, desired family size, spacing goal, and spacing effectiveness. The main finding is that given such modest family-size goals and provided that marriage age is young, the choice of narrow or wide spacing matters little with respect to the incidence of subfertility. Only when marriage is late and two or three children are wanted rather than one does the longer span of childbearing entailed by a wide-spacing goal materially augment the probability of not realizing the family-size objective.

The difference between a spacing effectiveness of .90 and 1.00 has little impact on the proportion subfertile, indicating that the results of Table 7.1 are rather insensitive to the choice of medium estimate of parameter e_s.

That the roles played by a bride's age at marriage, number of children

[4] An analysis of data collected in the *Princeton Fertility Study* puts the parameter e_s in the range of .81 to .83 (Westoff, Potter, Sagi and Mishler 1961, p. 100). From an analysis by Ryder (1973) of retrospective data corresponding to the 1950–1970 period, an e_s-estimate of .87 is derived (cf. Table 7.9). Both sources employed the concept of extended·use-effectiveness. Predicated on continuous practice of methods during the period 1970–1973, Vaughan *et al.* (1977) arrived at an average one-year use–failure rate of .073, implying an effectiveness e_s of .967. A corresponding failure rate measuring extended use-effectiveness is .125, implying an effectiveness e_s of .942. In this context, on grounds discussed in Footnote 2 of Chapter 8 and its related text, an effectiveness of .900 is interpreted as a low value corresponding roughly with, if not slightly underestimating, the extended use-effectiveness of coitus-related methods (ie., condom, diaphragm, foam, and rhythm) during the early 1970s.

Table 7.2
MEAN AGE OF WIFE AT BIRTH OF LAST DESIRED CHILD

Marriage age and number of children desired	No spacing	Medium spacing		Wide spacing	
		e = .90	e = 1.00	e = .90	e = 1.00
Marriage at age 20					
1 child desired	20.9	20.9	20.9	21.8	21.9
2 children	22.7	23.0	23.1	24.6	25.0
3 children	24.3	25.1	25.2	27.6	28.0
Marriage at age 25					
1 child desired	26.0	26.0	26.0	26.8	27.0
2 children	27.7	28.1	28.1	29.6	30.0
3 children	29.3	30.2	30.3	32.6	33.1
Marriage at age 30					
1 child desired	31.0	31.0	31.0	31.8	32.0
2 children	32.7	33.1	33.2	34.7	35.1
3 children	34.4	35.3	35.4	37.8	38.3

desired, spacing goal, and spacing effectiveness all depend on their contributing toward an earlier or later age of wife at last desired birth is confirmed by Table 7.2. In this table are given the mean ages of wife at attainment of desired family size among those achieving their family-size goal. A perfect rank correlation exists between the ages in Table 7.2 and the proportion subfertile in Table 7.1. Any combination of marriage age and family goals and spacing effectiveness that tend toward an older age at last desired birth works toward raising the proportion frustrated from having all the children they want by natural sterility.

The analysis based on REPMOD may be extended further. As compared to those couples who fail to reach desired family size, those who succeed are selected for higher natural fecundability and for better luck in terms of faster conception and less frequent pregnancy wastage than would be expected for their fecundity levels. The aggregate strength of these selections may be measured by considering how much lower is the average age at attainment of desired family size of those who succeed in the presence of natural sterility as compared to the mean potential age of those who failed.[5] That is, potential age is the age at which they would have attained desired family size had

[5] This extension of the analysis necessitates pairs of runs of REPMOD identical in every assumption except that one run includes the standard age schedule of onset of natural sterility whereas the other postpones sterility until some advanced age such as 49-years-old. Suppose that a proportion P attain desired family size in the first run at a mean age of $\overline{X}_1$. In the second run, with all couples attaining desired family size, the mean "potential" age of attainment is $\overline{X}$. The proportion P who succeeded in the first run command the same mean age of attainment $\overline{X}_1$ in the second run. Hence, the mean potential age of the $1 - P$ who failed must satisfy the equation $\overline{X}_2 = (\overline{X} - P\overline{X}_1)/(1 - P)$, since by definition, $\overline{X} = P\overline{X}_1 + (1 - P)\overline{X}_2$. A necessary condition for the analysis is that all couples attain their family-size goal in the second run that postpones sterility until an advanced age.

Table 7.3
PROPORTIONS FAILING TO REACH DESIRED FAMILY SIZE AMONG WIVES
MARRYING AT AGE 20 AND THEN TRYING TO DEFER CHILDBEARING FOR
10 YEARS

Number of children desired	Effectiveness of contraception [a]			
	e = .90		e = 1.00	
	Proportion failing	Mean age of attainment	Proportion failing	Mean age of attainment
1	.051	25.2	.088	31.0
2	.081	29.3	.110	32.7
3	.116	32.3	.147	34.4

[a] Effectiveness of contraception practiced in order to defer first birth. No effort to space subsequent children.

natural sterility been banished until some advanced age such as 49 years. Though not shown, a table comparable in scope to Tables 7.1 and 7.2 has been computed (but offering differences in mean age of attaining desired family size by those who do and mean potential age of attaining desired family size by those who do not). The differences prove trivially small, ranging from .00 to .23 (in years). The small magnitudes of these differences signifies that the predominant factor differentiating success and failure is not fecundity level or luck, but earliness of onset of natural sterility.

A case of special interest is that of a wife who marries at a young age, 20 years say, but to establish herself in her career, postpones childbearing until age 30, and then, to be out of the labor force as briefly as possible, forgoes contraception for spacing purposes. The proportion who will actually succeed in postponing their first born for 10 years depends on spacing effectiveness. Respecting the REPMOD runs summarized in Table 7.3, it is assumed that the couple react to a contraceptive failure not by resorting to induced abortion but by allowing the pregnancy to go to term, even if earlier than intended, and then pursuing a nonspacing goal with reference to any subsequent children wanted. It can be seen from Table 7.3 that given perfect spacing effectiveness, the proportions subfertile are the same as for couples from Table 7.1 who married at age 30 and wanted the same number of unspaced children. However, when spacing effectiveness is only .90, because of numerous contraceptive failures and attendant earlier childbearing, the proportion failing to attain desired family size is significantly reduced.

Simulations for Bangladesh

In Table 7.4, consideration shifts to a rural, third-world context represented by the simulation of the Bangladesh population in which postpartum anovulation is much longer, averaging 18.5 months, and this postpartum

Table 7.4

PROPORTION REACHING AND NOT REACHING DESIRED FAMILY SIZE AND
MEAN AGE OF WIFE AT ATTAINMENT, GIVEN MARRIAGE AGES AVERAGING
16.0 YEARS AND RELIANCE UPON POSTPARTUM ANOVULATION AVERAGING
18.5 MONTHS TO SPACE BIRTHS

Number pf children desired	Proportion failing	Reaching desired family size	
		Proportion succeeding	Mean age at attainment
2	.031	.969	20.8
3	.045	.955	23.8
4	.067	.933	26.8
5	.107	.893	29.7
6	.181	.819	32.4

infecundability rather than contraception is the basis of a much wider and
more highly variable birth spacing than would otherwise exist. A wider range
of desired family sizes are considered, from two to six children.

Age at marriage is made to conform to a Coale–McNeil curve with an
initial age of 11 and a mean age of 16 years. Indeed, the fecundity assumptions underlying Table 7.4 are exactly those of the first columns of Table 6.4
and 6.5, relating to natural fertility when no sources of variability are being
eliminated. Thanks to youthful marriage, the proportions failing to attain
their family-size objectives remain fairly low, under 10%, for goals of four
children or less. Among those succeeding in reaching these goals, the last

Table 7.5

PROPORTIONATE DISTRIBUTIONS OF NUMBERS OF CHILDREN NECESSARY
TO PRODUCE SPECIFIED NUMBERS OF SONS

Number of children	Intended number of sons		
	1	2	3
1	.512		
2	.250	.262	
3	.122	.256	.134
4	.059	.187	.196
5	.029	.122	.192
6	.014	.074	.156
7	.007	.044	.114
8	.003	.025	.078
9	.002	.014	.051
10	.002 [a]	.008	.032
11		.004	.019
12		.002	.011 [a]
13		.002 [a]	.017 [a]
Total	1.000	1.000	1.000

[a] Residual proportions

Table 7.6
PROPORTION FAILING TO ATTAIN DESIRED NUMBER OF SONS AND MEAN
AGE OF WIFE AT TIME OF LAST DESIRED SON, GIVEN A MARRIAGE AGE OF
16.0 AND POSTPARTUM ANOVULATION AVERAGING 18.5 MONTHS TO
SPACE BIRTHS

Number of desired sons	Reaching desired quota of sons		
	Proportion failing	Proportion succeeding	Mean age at attainment
1	.041	.959	20.5
2	.106	.894	26.2
3	.238	.762	31.3

desired birth is attained usually by the early thirties, if not the twenties, when the proportions sterile are still moderate. But with lengthy anovulation prolonging birth intervals, the proportion subfertile climbs to over 10% for a desired family size of five and approaches 20% when six children are wanted.

If the family-size objective is redefined as one, two, or three sons, the proportions fated for subfertility turn out higher than one might have anticipated. To see why, it is necessary first to ask how many children including daughters as well as sons do the couple need in order to reach their given quota of sons. As Table 7.5 documents, this number is highly variable, and when the number required is quite large, chances of not having all of them before natural sterility intervenes becomes appreciable.

The associated proportions subfertile are furnished in Table 7.6. For example, youthful marriage notwithstanding, achieving three sons is not at all assured inasmuch as the average number of births called for is almost six and an appreciable minority of couples require more than this number to have a third son. Note too that to have two sons implies having, on average, barely less than four children, but because there is so much variation in number of children required around this average, the proportion succeeding in having two sons is somewhat less than the proportion of success among couples simply seeking to have four children. This contrast in failure rates is .106 and .067. The difference is .041 to .031 between couples seeking respectively one son and two children regardless of sex composition; it is .238 to .181 between couples seeking three sons versus six children without regard to sex composition.

EXCESS FERTILITY

The calculations pertaining to subfertility have shown that if marriage is reasonably early, if the family goal does not involve a prolonged deferral of childbearing or exceed four children, and if the marriage remains intact until the wife reaches menopause, a great majority of the couples will eventually face a problem of preventing unwanted births.

In the discussion that occupies the rest of this chapter, excess fertility is treated as being determined by three sets of factors. First is the length of the risk period and the couple's fecundity during it. Second are the nature and efficiency of the couples' practice of family limitation. Involved here is continuity and effectiveness of contraception (including possibly a sterilizing operation) and willingness or not to resort to induced abortion. Third is the chance factor: Two alike couples with respect to the first two sets of factors may still experience quite different numbers of unintended births as a consequence of the host of small variables dictating whether or not a nonzero fecundability eventuates in conception during any month of exposure and whether a pregnancy, once conceived, spontaneously terminates.

If the couple are sterile at marriage, their risk period is 0. In the idealized conditions being assumed, namely, no divorce or separation and fixed family goals, a risk period starts with the attainment of desired family size and terminates with the onset of natural sterility or the sterilization of one of the partners. Here and in other connections, sterilization plays a special role. It approximates a contraceptive of perfect continuity and effectiveness. The approximation would be exact but for the temporary dangers of conception during the first few weeks following a vasectomy. Sterilization, whether of husband or wife, is usually abbreviating the risk period. By reducing fecundability to 0, it eliminates the play of chance factors. Indeed in the illustrations to follow pertaining to U.S. couples, sterilization is found to play a major role.

Length of Risk Period

When discussing the average length of risk period, two classes of couples must be distinguished. First are the couples who prove their nonsterility at some age x by the wife having her last desired birth at that age. The possibility of an onset of sterility at ages younger than x is excluded. As a result, for these couples, mean age at onset of natural sterility must necessarily exceed the average of 41.7 years estimated for couples taken at random from the population. It is shown in Table 7.7, predicated on the age schedule of natural sterility of Henry (1965), that as wife's age at last desired birth increases, her expected mean age at onset of natural sterility also increases, which means that her average length of risk period decreases more slowly than would otherwise be the case.

Second are the newlyweds wishing no children. For them, the probabilities of being sterile already and therefore enjoying 0 risk periods are (Henry 1965) .03, .05, .08, .15, and .32 at ages 20, 25, 30, 35, and 40, respectively.

Table 7.7
AVERAGE LENGTH OF RISK PERIOD ACCORDING TO AGE OF WIFE UPON
ATTAINING DESIRED FAMILY SIZE OR AT TIME OF MARRIAGE WHEN WISHING
NO CHILDREN

| Age of Wife | Mean length of risk period | | Mean age at onset of natural sterility [a] |
	At marriage	At last desired birth	
20	21.0	21.7	41.7
25	16.2	17.1	42.1
30	11.6	12.6	42.6
35	7.1	8.4	43.4
40	3.3	4.8	44.8

[a] Mean age among wives sharing a specified age at last desired birth.

Their overall mean length of risk period (first column of Table 7.7) are reduced by these proportions as compared to mothers reaching their family-
size objectives at corresponding ages (second column of Table 7.7).[6]

It is to be kept in mind that chances of an unwanted birth are not constant
during risk periods. Approaching menopause, natural fecundability is relatively low and the risk of spontaneous pregnancy wastage is relatively high.
As one moves back toward earlier ages, rates of potential natural fertility
rise. Consequently, in the absence of contraception and induced abortion,
the expected number of excess births increases disproportionately with
length of risk period. However, as demonstrated by Table 7.8, these dispro-
portionalities prove modest in the simulated Bangladesh and U.S. populations. The rise in average potential fertility consequent on an earlier start of
the risk period is measured by dividing total excess births expected in the
absence of family limitation by the average length of the risk period. The rise
is so gradual because gestation lengths and postpartum infecundability stay
constant, whereas only natural fecundability and risk of spontaneous abor-

[6] The results of Table 7.7 are derived as follows. Let the proportion still fecund at age x in a
population be denoted $f(x)$ and the proportion becoming sterile between exact ages x and $x + 1$
(x is an integer in years) be designated by $s(x) = f(x) - f(x + 1)$. Assume a uniform distribution
of sterility onsets over any year of age. Then the mean length of risk period, $R(x_0)$, if desired
family size is attained at integral age x_0 becomes

$$R(x_0) = \sum_{x=x_0}^{49} s(x)(x + 0.5)/f(x_0).$$

Respecting a couple married at age x_0 and wishing no children, as their fertility at age x_0 is
untested, their chance of being already sterile and therefore possessing a 0 risk period is $1 -
f(x_0)$. If not sterile at marriage, their mean length of risk period is $R(x_0)$, computed as above.
Taken over both contingencies, their expected length of risk period is $f(x_0)R(x_0)$.

Table 7.8

MEAN ANNUAL PROBABILITY OF A BIRTH IN THE ABSENCE OF FAMILY
LIMITATION, BY AGE AT START OF RISK PERIOD

Age at attainment of desired family size	Corresponding length of risk period a/	United States context b/		Bangladesh context c/	
		Total excess births	Mean annual excess births	Total excess births	annual excess births
20	21.7	11.53	.53	6.53	.30
25	17.1	8.94	.52	5.17	.30
30	12.6	6.04	.48	3.64	.29
35	8.4	3.47	.41	2.23	.27

a/ Taken from second column of Table 7.7.

b/ Mean plateau fecundability of .19 and mean postpartum anovulation of
    3.0 months.

c/ Mean plateau fecundability of .16 and mean postpartum anovulation of
    18.5 months.

tion change with age. The sensitivity of average potential fertility to age at
start of the risk period is less for Bangladesh than the United States because
the fixed average length of anovulation is 18.5 months instead of 3.0 and
therefore a major component of birth intervals at any age of the wife. Clearly
any delaying of the start of the risk period enhances control over family size
mainly by shortening the risk period and only very secondarily by reducing
the average level of potential natural fertility during it.

Effectiveness of Contraception

How far contraception reduces fertility depends on how continuously it is
practiced and how completely, when practiced, it lowers natural fecundability. Equally important, then, are the two aspects of continuation and effectiveness. Different contraceptives vary widely in both their continuation
rates and effectiveness. Any class of contraceptives—IUD, pill, condom,
foam, diaphragm, or rhythm—is practiced with varying efficiency in different
populations and even by the same sample of couples at different stages of
their reproductive careers. As remarked already, it is well documented that
couples seeking to delay eventually desired births practice contraception less
assiduously than couples seeking to prevent unwanted births.

Properties such as residual fecundability, continuation rates, natural
fecundability, and contraceptive effectiveness cannot be measured for individual couples, but only measured, more or less indirectly, for samples of
couples. Discontinuation rates refer to the cumulative proportions becoming

pregnant or discontinuing for other reasons during a segment confined to the practice of a single, identified method. For present purposes, more relevant are cumulative-use–failure rates, defined in Chapter 3, representing the cumulative proportions pregnant among women who practice a specified method without discontinuation, except for reason of accidental pregnancy. A lifetable methodology is necessary in order to avoid the biases that would accrue from so many segments of contraception being censored by end of observation, discontinuation for reason other than accidental pregnancy, or loss to follow-up. Affecting the cumulative proportions pregnant are the couples' natural fecundabilities as well as the effectiveness of their contraceptive method. Given in the bottom panel of Table 7.9 are the 12-month use–failure rates classified by method and reproductive intent from Vaughan, Trussell, Menken, and Jones (1977) for a national sample of ever-married couples of the United States, based on the 1973 *National Survey of Family Growth*. The main report of these important results is found in Vaughan *et al.* (1977) with additional commentary in Menken, Trussell, Ford

Table 7.9

PERCENTAGE OF MARRIED COUPLES WHO FAIL TO DELAY THEIR WANTED NEXT PREGNANCY OR TO PREVENT AN UNWANTED PREGNANCY AND IMPLIED EFFECTIVENESS OF CONTRACEPTION, BY INTENTION, METHODOLOGY, AND METHOD

Method and methodology	Percentage failing to delay	Implied effectiveness[b]	Percentage failing to prevent	Implied effectiveness[c]
	Estimates of Ryder (1973)			
Extended use effectiveness:				
pill	7	.968	4	.976
IUD	15	.929	5	.969
condom	21	.897	10	.937
diaphragm	25	.875	17	.889
foam	36	.807	22	.853
rhythm	38	.794	21	.860
all methods [a]	26	.869	14	.904
	Estimates of Vaughan, Trussell, Menken and Jones (1977)			
Use-effectiveness:				
pill	2.0	.991	2.0	.988
IUD	5.6	.975	2.9	.982
condom	13.7	.935	6.6	.959
diaphragm	15.9	.924	10.3	.934
foam	16.7	.920	13.1	.918
rhythm	28.8	.852	9.5	.941
all methods [a]	7.3	.967	3.7	.976

[a] Including sterilization.

[b] Based on a natural fecundability of .19.

[c] Predicated on a natural fecundability of .14 for individual methods, and .13 for all methods including sterilization.

and Pratt (1979) and Trussell and Menken (1981). The sizeable contrasts among methods are manifest as well as the responsiveness of the failure rate to contraceptive motive, (i.e., delaying versus preventing pregnancy).

In a modern setting, with many different methods available, it is commonplace for couples to switch from one method to another. A single pregnancy interval may include use of two or more methods, sometimes punctuated by a subinterval of nonuse. This complexity of practice, and the attendant problems of measurement, have led to the concept of extended use–failure rates (Tietze and Lewit 1973), by which is meant cumulative proportions pregnant during a pregnancy inerval, identified by the first method employed and usually also by contraceptive incentive, delaying or preventing. When the object is to compare contraceptives, pregnancy intervals are typically restricted to those in which a single method is reported. An example are the 12-month extended-use–failure rates occupying the top panel of Table 7.9. Derived by Ryder (1973), these rates are based on the 1970 *National Fertility Study*. Again, wide contrasts among methods are found along with differentiation by reproductive intent. Not surprisingly, the cumulative proportions pregnant at the end of specified durations tend to be appreciably higher on account of the intermittent rather than continuous practice of the method in question.

The analysis of Trussell and Menken (1981) permits one to derive an extended-use–failure rate for all methods combined (including sterilization) among preventers during the 1970–1973 period. This 1-year failure rate turns out to be .051,[7] roughly a third of the corresponding rate of .14 derived by Ryder (1973) for the earlier 1950–1970 epoch. Contributing to the large difference are the more favorable mix of methods practiced as well as the higher extended use-effectiveness of individual methods prevailing in the 1970–1973 period as compared to the earlier 1950–1970 era.

Also derivable from the analysis of Trussell and Menken (1981) is a 12-month extended-use–failure rate of .064 for all methods combined excluding sterilization.

To estimate the average effectiveness of a method being practiced by a sample of couples, $1 - f_r/f_n$, the first step is to convert a failure rate, usually a 12-month failure rate, into a measure of mean residual fecundability f_r. The most convenient formula for this purpose is that of Equation (12) of Chapter

---

[7] With respect to preventers, Trussell and Menken (1981) report 1-year use–failure rates for all methods combined, including sterilization, separately for whites and blacks. What are needed for present purposes are an extended-use–failure rate for all methods combined and one for all nonpermanent methods combined, but neither rate subdivided by race. To achieve this, their formula $P_e = P_u C + (1 - C)f_n$ for converting P_u, the complement of a cumulative use–failure rate, into P_e, the complement of a cumulative extended-use–failure rate, is employed. The symbol C denotes a 1-year continuation rate when the only source of attrition is stopping contraception. P_n signifies the conditional probability of not becoming pregnant given that contraception was abandoned in the particular pattern observed over the course of the first year. When averaging the two racial groups, coefficients associated with whites are weighted .9; those associated with blacks are weighted .1.

3, namely, $f_r = 1 - F/12f_n(1 - 0.5F)$, F being the given failure rate. As explained in the Appendix of Chapter 3, Equation (12) gives results that are virtually identical with those obtained by taking the inverse of a formula popularized by Ryder (1973).[8] The latter explicitly assumes homogeneity among couples. Because heterogeneity exists, with couples varying in natural fecundability as well as both continuation and effectiveness of contraception, the conversion tends to underestimate f_r and therefore to overestimate effectiveness e. However unless effectiveness is below .8, the distortion is not likely to be large and becomes smaller and smaller as effectiveness approaches 1.0.[9] The conversions of 12-month failure rates into contraceptive effectiveness, in Table 7.9, are based on Formula (12) combined with a natural fecundability f_n of .19 among delayers and of .13 or .14 among birth preventers.[10]

A fundamental question is whether an effectiveness of contraception consistent with empirical estimates yields the kind of protection against excess fertility being claimed in interview surveys. Ostensible success at family limitation among U.S. couples has steadily improved over the time span for which there have been national surveys. For the period 1975–1976, the fraction of all pregnancies classified as unwanted is 9%, down from 12% for 1970–1973, figures to be compared with 14% for 1966–1970 and 24% for

---

[8] Ryder's formula is $F = 1 - (1 - f_r)^{12}$, from which, noting that $f_r = (1 - e)f_n$, $e = 1 - (1 - \exp(C)/f_n)$ with $C = \ln(1 - F)/12$. In application to Table 7.9, upper panel, the two formulas, Ryder's and Formula (12) from Chapter 3, generate values of e that differ at most by 1.0 in the third decimal place. Virtually identical with the other, Formula (12) is favored only for its convenience of calculation.

[9] In terms of the argument given in the Appendix of Chapter 3, high contraceptive effectiveness means that $P(n)$ terms remain small and $f(n)$ terms relatively invariant, conditions for the more general formulas encompassing heterogeneity to yield results close to those representing homogeneity.

[10] The estimate of $f_n = .14$ for family limiters using a nonpermanent method in the 1970–1973 period entails a less simple calculation dictated by the following considerations.

1. Equal emphasis upon medium- and wide-spacing goals, combined with an average desired family size of two children and an average age at first marriage of 22 years, leads to a mean age at last wanted birth of approximately 26 years. Accordingly for those couples who never obtain a sterilization and who practice contraception to prevent births between average age limits of 26 and 45 years, mean fecundability averages out to be .13.

2. From statistics provided by Menken *et al.* (1979), prevalence of sterilization among preventers may be put at about .20.

3. A distribution of intervals from last wanted birth to sterilizing operation is provided by Westoff and McCarthy (1979); this distribution, combined with a mean age of mother at last wanted birth of 26, defines the ages at which nonpermanent contraception is being practiced to prevent births by those couples who eventually obtained a sterilization. These ages are young enough to make a f_n-estimate of .17 appropriate.

4. Weighting .17 and .13 by .20 and .80 produces an overall estimate of .14, the value assigned to f_n for preventers using individual nonpermanent methods in the lower panel of Table 7.9. For all methods combined, including sterilization, among preventers, a f_n-value of .13 is adopted. These same values of average f_n are applied to the 1950–1970 period as well.

1961–1965 (Anderson, 1981). More relevant are the implied cumulative numbers of unwanted births per couple if the rates specific to each year of marriage duration from last desired birth for a calendar period are summed. Westoff (1981) performed this calculation and estimated a cumulative average excess fertility rate of .38 for the 1971–1973 synthetic cohort and .20 for the 1974–1976 cohort, based on the 30-month experiences preceding the 1973 and 1976 NSFG Surveys.

Naturally these estimates are not to be accepted at face value. It has not proven feasible to secure useful responses about induced abortion in the two national fertility surveys. Statistics from the Center of Disease Control, cited by Tietze (1981), indicate a total induced abortion rate of about .1 for married U.S. women of the 1970–1973 period. Presumably most of these abortions are motivated by unwanted rather than mistimed pregnancies. The frequency of .10 added to .38 lifts the conjectured per couple frequency of unwanted pregnancies for the 1970–1973 period to about the .50 level. Furthermore, as Menken *et al.* (1979) have stressed, many pregnancies originally unwanted but not deliberately interrupted are soon accommodated to, and subsequently reported as wanted, even if mistimed. It is difficult to gauge the frequency of this class of pregnancies.

The requirements for three standards of protection will be explored by means of REPMOD. These standards are averages of .20, .38, and .50 for excess births per couple attaining desired family size and eschewing induced abortion. The most stringent standard of .20 corresponds to what was claimed by couples in the mid-seventies. The medium standard of .38 represents the counterpart for the early 1970s. The relatively lax standard of .50 excess births per couple may approximate roughly the mean number of originally unwanted births by couples of the 1970–1973 period, that is, including the potential births prevented by deliberate abortion, the rationalized births, and finally the births frankly acknowledged as unwanted.

It will be shown that without sterilization, nonpermanent contraception and the average levels of effectiveness reported would require a heavy supplement of induced abortion in order to account for the level of protection being claimed by survey respondents. However, with sterilization included, something closer to a consistency among various estimates is won. For this analysis, a special version of REPMOD is required.[11]

---

[11] Another adaptation of REPMOD is needed to stimulate couples who attain desired famiy size at a common age Y (in years) and from that age onward seek to avoid additional pregnancies. If A is the average length of postpartum anovulation, these couples reach the end of the postpartum anovulatory period following the last desired birth at mean age $Y + A$. To represent experience during the risk period, "marriage" is set at age $Y + A$ and desired famiy size is made 0 as no more children are wanted. Therefore, fecundability, subject to contraception practiced for limiting purposes, becomes $f_r(a) = (1 - e_1)f_n(a)$. Depending on whether contraception is being backstopped or not by induced abortion, either no pregnancies or all pregnancies surviving into the third month of gestation are terminated. Mean final parity is interpreted as mean

Calibre of Family Limitation

NONPERMANENT CONTRACEPTION AND ABORTION

Let us start with an exclusive reliance on nonpermanent contraception of specified effectiveness by couples attaining desired family size at given ages. Based on the concept of extended use-effectiveness, an average 1-year failure rate of .064 was obtained for the 1970–1973 period. This coefficient converts into a limiting effectiveness of .958 when a natural fecundability of .13 is postulated. Based on runs of REPMOD, mean numbers and standard deviations of unwanted births consequent upon a total reliance on contraception taken at five different values of effectiveness within the range of .800 and .975 for couples attaining desired famiy size at 25, 30, or 35 years of age, or else marrying at age 20 and wanting no children, are presented in Table 7.10.

For a given limiting effectiveness, the mean number of unwanted births climbs rapidly, the earlier the family-size goal is attained. If the last wanted child comes when the mother is only age 25, a limiting effectiveness higher than .975 is necessary to reach a relatively lax standard of .5 excess births per couple. Even when the risk period does not start until age 30, a limiting effectiveness above .95 is needed for this calibre of protection.

Values of contraception effectiveness of .80 or higher connote low residual fecundabilities. That the expected numbers of unwanted births in Table 7.10 are so high is explained by the long lengths of risk period, which translate into many months of risk of contraceptive failure. To take a single example, if a given couple are practicing contraception at 95% effectiveness, their residual fecundability might start at $f_r = (1 - e_s)f_n = .05(.19) = .0095$, less than .01, seemingly a very low monthly probability of conception and decline thereafter with increasing age. However, if the risk period is starting when the mother is aged 30, its average length of 12.6 years (cf. Table 7.7) implies about 150 monthly trials when accidental pregnancy is risked.

Another interesting result is the very large variation in numbers of unwanted births from couple to couple around respective means. Many of the standard deviations exceed the corresponding means. Such great variability in excess fertility is attributable to the sizable variability in length of risk period, heterogeneity of fecundability, and the play of chance factors.

---

excess births, and correspondingly for the standard deviation. One minus the proportion reaching parity one yields the proportion escaping excess fertility.

One further adjustment remains. One has to modify the age schedule at onset of natural sterility to reflect continued nonsterility up to age Y. As before, let the proportion of the entire population fertile at age x be denoted $f(x)$, x measured in integral years, and $s(x) = f(x) - f(x + 1)$. With $f(50) = 0$, $\sum_{x=Y}^{49} s(x) = f(Y)$. We want a set of adjusted proportions becoming sterile between exact ages x to $x + 1$, $s^*(x)$, which over age-range Y to 49 will sum to 1.0 and thereby assure a proper probability distribution function. Satisfying this requirement is

$$s^*(x) = s(x)/f(Y) \qquad x = Y, Y + 1, \ldots, 49.$$

Table 7.10
MEAN μ AND STANDARD DEVIATION σ OF EXCESS BIRTHS WHEN CONTRACEPTION
ALONE IS USED, BY EFFECTIVENESS OF THAT CONTRACEPTION AND AGE WHEN
FAMILY SIZE GOAL IS REACHED

Effectiveness of contraception	Newly wed: aged 20		Age of parents at time of last desired birth					
			25		30		35	
	μ	σ	μ	σ	μ	σ	μ	σ
.80	4.64	2.52	3.49	1.97	2.22	1.51	1.15	1.07
.85	3.73	2.22	2.79	1.75	1.76	1.35	.90	.95
.90	2.69	1.83	2.00	1.47	1.25	1.13	.63	.79
.95	1.46	1.30	1.08	1.07	.67	.82	.33	.57
.975	.77	.91	.57	.76	.35	.59	.17	.41

To make more vivid just how variable is unwanted fertility from couple to
couple when nonpermanent contraception of constant limiting effectiveness
is being relied upon exclusively, Table 7.11 presents the probability distributions of unwanted births for five values of limiting effectiveness, given
women whose risk periods commence at age 30. The highest probability in
each distribution is underlined. It is apparent from this table that the unsatisfactoriness of a strategy that relies wholly on nonpermanent contraception is
not merely the high mean number of unsought births whenever limiting
effectiveness fails to be very high but the fact that a nontrivial minority will
exceed the modal number of unwanted births by two or more. Obviously
too, the problem is accentuated when the mother has her last wanted birth at
an earlier age, such as 25-years-old.

What are the values of limiting effectiveness (taken to three decimal
places) that come closest to realizing the three standards of protection defined earlier, given specified ages at start of the risk period? These levels of
effectiveness are given in Table 7.12, derived iteratively by means of
REPMOD. For risk periods beginning at 25 years of age, achievement of a

Table 7.11
NUMBER OF UNWANTED BIRTHS WHEN NONPERMANENT CONTRACEPTION
ALONE IS USED, BY EFFECTIVENESS OF THAT CONTRACEPTION, MOTHERS
STARTING THEIR RISK PERIODS AT AGE 30

Effectiveness of contraception	Number of unwanted children									Mean number
	0	1	2	3	4	5	6	7	8	
.80	.125	.233	.248	.196	.119	.055	.018	.004	.001	2.22
.85	.187	.288	.254	.161	.076	.026	.006	.001		1.76
.90	.297	.343	.221	.099	.031	.007	.001			1.25
.95	.517	.335	.117	.027	.004					.67
.975	.708	.243	.044	.005						.35

Table 7.12

EFFECTIVENESS OF CONTRACEPTION NECESSARY FOR SPECIFIED STANDARDS OF FAMILY LIMITATION, AND ATTENDANT STANDARD DEVIATIONS IN NUMBERS OF UNWANTED BIRTHS (IN PARENTHESES), WHEN CONTRACEPTION IS USED ALONE, BY AGE WHEN FAMILY SIZE GOAL IS REACHED

Per capita number of excess births	Newlywed aged 20	Age of parents when family goal is reached		
		25	30	35
.50	.984 (.73)	.978 (.72)	.963 (.71)	.922 (.71)
.38	.988 (.63)	.983 (.63)	.972 (.62)	.943 (.61)
.20	.994 (.44)	.991 (.46)	.986 (.45)	.970 (.45)

medium standard of protection (.38 excess births per couple) requires a limiting effectiveness of .983, a value which, according to the Vaughan *et al.* estimates (Table 7.9), is higher than the use-effectiveness of any nonpermanent method except the pill. Requirements are even higher for those marrying at age 20 and intending no children. On the other hand, prerequisites decline as start of the risk period is made later. For instance, the estimate of average extended use-effectiveness of .958 suffices for a medium standard of protection when desired family size is not attained until age 35, but it is not quite adequate to reach the same standard if the risk period begins at 30.

Even if specific standards of protection are being achieved thanks to contraception of exactly the appropriate effectiveness, there still exists the disadvantage of a very large variation of individually experienced excess fertility around the mean defining the standard. The standard deviations measuring this variability appear in parentheses besides the corresponding coefficient of limiting effectiveness.

The futility of a strategy that depends exclusively on repeated abortion and employs no contraception is made clear by a single example. Wives who reach their family-size goal at age 30, if they practice no contraception, would have to average 11.73 induced abortions, according to the appropriate run of REPMOD, in order to hold unwanted births at 0. This does not count the 8 or 9% of pregnancies ending in recognized spontaneous wastage early enough to obviate an abortion procedure. And of course there would be a huge spread in the numbers of induced abortions from couple to couple around the appalling mean of 11.73. Moreover, high as it is, this mean of 11.73 would be augmented by 5.0 or more if the family-size goal were attained at age 25 instead of 30.

A third, idealized strategy that can be simulated by REPMOD is nonpermanent contraception of constant effectiveness, backed by induced abortion. The number of induced abortions required to hold unwanted births to 0 proves appreciably higher than the expected number of births, given no

Table 7.13
MEAN NUMBER OF INDUCED, SPONTANEOUS, AND TOTAL ABORTIONS, AND
POTENTIAL UNWANTED BIRTHS, BY EFFECTIVENESS OF CONTRACEPTION,
GIVEN A LAST DESIRED BIRTH AT AGE 30

Effectiveness of contraception	Mean number of abortions			Potential ratios of	
	Induced	Spontaneous	Total	Unwanted births	Induced abortions to births
.00	11.73	1.00	12.73	6.04	1.94
.80	3.10	.26	3.36	2.22	1.40
.85	2.37	.20	2.57	1.76	1.35
.90	1.62	.14	1.76	1.25	1.30
.95	.83	.07	.90	.67	1.24

deliberate interruptions of pregnancy and the same effectiveness of contraception. Table 7.13 provides five comparisons of contraception with and
without an abortion backup. The ratio between number of induced abortions
and live births prevented grows progressively less favorable, the less effective is contraception.

The unfavorable ratio depends on two factors. A fraction of the pregnancies deliberately interrupted would have ended in spontaneous loss any-
way.[12] Second and more important, given the modern context being depicted, interruption of a pregnancy that might have ended in a live birth
involves forfeiting an average of 6 months of gestation and 3 months of
postpartum anovulation, thereby increasing to that extent the number of
fecundable exposure months when additional pregnancies are a possibility.
Moreover, there still remains the serious problem that individual couples
experience a great variation in number of induced abortions around the
mean, implying intolerable abortion loads for the unlucky minority.

STERILIZATION

With sterilization included, the 1-year extended use–failure rate among
preventers derived for the 1970–1973 period was .051, a reduction of .013
from the corresponding rate for nonpermanent methods alone. This lower

[12] This factor by itself implies a ratio of about 112 induced abortions per 100 potential births.
In the absence of induced abortion, given a probability of .17 that any pregnancy ends spontaneously in wastage, $(1.00 + .17/.83)100 = 122$ pregnancies are required to produce 100 live births.
In Table 7.13 it is assumed that half of all pregnancies fated for spontaneous wastage will
terminate by natural causes early enough to obviate an abortion procedure. It follows that
among couples determined not to let any pregnancy go to term, corresponding to 100 potential
births are $(.085)122 = 10.4$ spontaneous abortions and $(.915)122 = 111.6$ induced abortions.

failure rate translates into an average effectiveness of .966. Looking again at Table 7.12, one sees that this effectiveness is somewhat below the requirement of .972 for meeting the medium standard of family limitation (.38 excess births) when family size is attained at age 30 or the requirement of .978 to meet the relatively more lax standard of .50 excess births when the last wanted birth occurs at age 25.

A reason for believing that .966 may be an underestimate of average limiting effectiveness is that it is derived from a first-year extended use–failure rate. Not given any weight in the calculation are the failure rates at higher durations, which tend to be appreciably lower. For example, Trussell and Menken (1981) reported a second-year use–failure rate for all methods combined that is one-third lower than the first year counterpart, .033 as compared to .051. (With sterilization included, the decline is from .037 to .024.) If the second-year rate of .033 is interpreted as more representative than the first year rate of .051, then one is dealing with an implied limiting effectiveness of .978, a level which comes very close to meeting the medium standard of protection for risk periods starting as early as age 25 years.

SOME ADDITIONAL TOPICS

Three additional topics have been explored by means of the macrosimulation REPMOD. In deference to an already long chapter, these results will be summarized rather than the full details presented.

Timing of Excess Births

As the effectiveness of contraception is enhanced, the proportion of couples escaping excess fertility is augmented, but among those who experience at least one unwanted birth the proportion who do so after an inconveniently long interval, such as 5 or more years after the last desired birth, goes up too. For example, given a limiting effectiveness of .98, among wives reaching desired family size at age 30 and subsequently having an unwanted birth, the proportion who experience that event 5 or more years later is calculated from a relevant run of REPMOD as 48%. This proportion climbs the higher contraceptive effectiveness is or the earlier the attainment of desired family size is.

An explanation is readily attained by appeal to the geometric distribution.[13] This distribution, predicated on a constant monthly probability of con-

---

[13] The phenomenon in question follows from the properties of the geometric distribution. Suppose that residual fecundability, denoted by f_r, remains constant from month to month and that the length of risk period R exceeds 5 years. Under these conditions, the expected propor-

traceptive failure in an unlimited reproductive period, demonstrates that as the monthly risk is reduced, the scatter of waiting times to failure increases, which means a smaller and smaller proportion of all failures within any given initial interval such as 4 or 5 years. Both the presence of natural sterility and the gradual declining of natural fecundability with aging tend to dilute this effect but not very much if desired family size is being realized as early as age 30 years.

Premarital Conceptions

Another issue of present-day importance is the increased difficulties of successful family limitation when a premarital conception precipitates an unintended marriage. Such involuntary marriages may become common again if current efforts to make induced abortion less accessible to American women succeed. By making marriage earlier and by shortening the interval from marriage to first birth, the unscheduled pregnancy tends to prolong the risk period and to assure a higher fecundity during it.

Illustrating consequences are a set of REPMOD runs representing three control groups who marry at 20 years and want two children spaced according to close, medium, or wide master schedules. Each of these three groups are compared with couples having the same preferred interval between the two desired children but whose marriages are precipitated at specified ages younger than 20, and followed 3 months later by the first birth.[14] Limiting effectiveness is set at a value of .95, and for those pursuing a medium or wide master schedule spacing goal, spacing effectiveness is fixed at .90.

To take an example, a couple whose marriage takes place 2.5 years earlier, at age 17.5, supposedly have their first birth at age 17.75, which compares with expected ages at first birth among the control couples of 21.5, 21.5, and

---

tion escaping excess fertility is $(1 - f_r)^{12R}$, a fraction that plainly increases as f_r is made lower. The expected ratio of first unwanted conceptions in ordinal month of exposure $x + 1$ to those in ordinal exposure month x is given by $(1 - f_r)^x f_r/(1 - f_r)^{x-1} f_r = (1 - f_r)$. Clearly this ratio approaches 1.0 as f_r is reduced toward 0. Thus a residual fecundity close enough to 0 yields an approximately uniform distribution of waiting times to conception, of which, to the same approximation, an expected fraction $5/R$ will be less than 5 years in duration and $(R-5)/R$ longer than 5 years.

[14] REPMOD is easily modified to represent couples desiring two children, but with the first born arriving 3 months after marriage, at age $y - 1/4$ say. Whereas marriage is interpreted as having taken place at age $y - 1/2$, the REPMOD parameter for marriage age is set at the expected time when the wife recovers fecundable status after her first birth. The parameter of desired family size is reduced to 1.0, as only one additional birth is wanted after the first, and the parameter MB, which now represents the intended interval between first and second birth, is set at 12, 24, or 36 months depending on whether the master schedule goal is close, medium, or wide. To reflect the absence of sterility prior to age $y - 1/4$, the proportions fecund at specified ages older than $y - 1/4$, from Henry (1965), are inflated by a factor of $(.98)^{-1} = 1.02$.

22.5 years, depending on their spacing goal. These contrasts in ages at first birth, ranging from 3.75 to 4.75 years, translate into virtually equivalent lengthenings of risk period, which produce .37–.45 additional excess births per couple. Stated otherwise, within the range of examples considered, each year of risk period added produces from .07 to .09 additional unwanted births.

Not registered in these illustrative calculations are the indirect or selective effects. Empirical research has shown that girls who have premarital conceptions tend to be selected in ways that make them less efficient contraceptors than average. These selectivities may be quite as important as the direct effects just illustrated when it comes to their inferior records as family limiters. Also being neglected are the qualifying roles placed by induced abortion and sterilization. Owing to deliberate interruptions of pregnancy, a premarital conception frequently does not precipitate a marriage. To the extent that premarital conception does hasten marriage and lengthen risk periods, it increases chances of at least one excess birth, which, in turn, according to a differential adduced by Westoff and McCarthy (1979), inflates the probability of a sterilizing operation before the end of the reproductive period.

Lower Potential Fertility

A third topic requires widening the setting to include rural Bangladesh as well as the United States. How much does longer postpartum anovulation, averaging 18.5 instead of 3.0 months, help toward reducing excess fertility for a given effectiveness of contraception. The answer, a little startling at first, makes sense on reflection. Much longer postpartum anovulation makes a big difference in the absence of contraception or when it is inefficient, but as contraception is made more and more effective, the presence of prolonged postpartum infecundability becomes an increasingly minor factor.

For example, according to simulation results based on risk periods commencing at age 30, the difference in expected excess births per couple between wives having fecundity parameters representative of contemporary United States and those representative of present-day rural Bangladesh depends as follows on level of contraceptive effectiveness: for effectiveness 0 (i.e., no contraception) the expected difference in excess births is 2.40 per couple; with an effectiveness of .90, that difference slips to .29 per couple; while an effectiveness of .95 reduces the difference to only .13 excess births per couple.

The reason for this drastic shrinking of effect from prolonged postpartum infecundability is not far in seeking. If effective contraception is permitting few births, then it matters little whether postpartum anovulation is short or long; there will be relatively few postpartum infecundable months per risk period in either case. For example, contraception effective enough to confer a medium standard of protection because it permits only an average of .38 excess births per risk period allows, at the same time, only an average of about 7 months of anovulation in the Bangladesh case and 1 month in the U.S. example. For risk periods averaging 12.6 years or longer (equivalent to starting ages of 30 years or younger), a half-year difference in months held infecundable by anovulation does not constitute a major influence.

SUMMARY

Family-size control has two main aspects: attaining the number of children desired and holding family size to that level. Subfertility constitutes a failure to achieve the first objective. When youthful marriage combines with modest family-size aspirations to assure that the mother potentially completes her childbearing before age 30, the proportion subfertile remains well below 10%. Under these conditions, whether or not the couple deliberately space their desired births, and thereby prolong intervals between consecutive children by 1 or 2 years, has little influence on the fraction subfertile. Only when marriage age approaches 30, and two or three children are wanted rather than one, do spacing goals appreciably differentiate the incidence of subfertility.

Interestingly enough, the incidence of subfertility associated with seeking a specified number of boys (or a predesignated number of girls) is non-trivially higher than the subfertility associated with the goal of having twice that number of children but without regard to sex composition. This inequality arises from the large chance variation in the number of sons and daughters required to reach a given number of children of the same sex.

The combination of youthful marriage and modest family-size goal, which reduces the risk of subfertility thanks to a relatively early completion of desired childbearing, at the same time increases the length of the "risk period" from attainment of desired family size to onset of sterility, and consequently contributes to excess fertility. In a series of REPMOD runs simulating modern conditions, risk-period length is explored in relation to marriage age, number of children wanted, spacing goals, and effectiveness of contraception employed for spacing purposes. A point easily overlooked is that, as the age of the mother upon attainment of desired family size increases, length of risk period decreases less than proportionally because the average age at onset of secondary sterility goes up. The very occurrence of a later last birth is selecting against an early episode of natural sterility and thereby contributes to a higher average age at end of reproductive capacity.

Respecting excess fertility, three standards of family limitation were investigated by means of REPMOD in a U.S. context. These standards involve averages of .20, .38, and .50 excess births per couple whose first marriage remained intact until past menopause. The most demanding standard of .20

corresponds to what was claimed by married respondents in the middle 1970s. The medium standard of .38 constituted the counterpart for the early 1970s. The more lax standard of .50 excess births per couple represents an upward adjustment of the latter in order to encompass the estimated incidence of induced abortion and associated unreported accidental pregnancies. The levels of contraceptive effectiveness required to reach these standards when contraception alone is being relied upon for protection are assessed in relation to specified ages at last desired birth. The required levels of effectiveness of nonpermanent methods prove dauntingly high, well above the average level of extended use-effectiveness reported for U.S. couples. Then too, a strategy of exclusive reliance on induced abortion may be dismissed at once for implying wholly implausible numbers of operations to hold down excess fertility to criterion values. What essentially accounts for the calibre of family limitation claimed by U.S. couples in nationally representative interview surveys is the combination of contraception, induced abortion, and sterilization taken at respective average values.

Three further issues were addressed, two of them applicable to the U.S. setting. First, assuming that induced abortion is eschewed, highly efficient contraception can be counted on to lower the fraction of family limiters who suffer an unwanted birth, but unfortunately that same highly efficient contraception also raises the likelihood of an inconveniently long interval to any first unwanted birth that does occur. Secondly, when a marriage is precipitated by a premarital conception allowed to go to term, the risk period is augmented, with a correspondingly higher expectation of excess fertility. The size of this increment in excess fertility under specified conditions has been indicated.

The Bangaldesh context was invoked in order to demonstrate a final point. Prolonged, as opposed to brief postpartum anovulation, significantly reduces fertility when contraception is absent or at least inefficient. But when highly effective contraception is practiced by family limiters, so few pregnancies are allowed to happen that length of postpartum anovulation, which after all depends for its existence on parturition, becomes almost irrelevant. Stated otherwise, the calibre of contraception necessary to attain a high standard of family limitation is not really eased at all by the presence of lengthy anovulation following childbirth.

REFERENCES

Anderson, J. E. (1981), "Planned and Unplanned Births in the United States: 1. Planning Status of Marital Births, 1975–1976," *Family Planning Perspectives, 13,* 2 (March/April), 62–70.

Bongaarts, J. (1978), "A Framework for Analyzing the Proximate Determinants of Fertility," *Population and Development Review, 4,* 1 (March), 103–132.

Bongaarts, J. (1980), The Fertility Inhibiting Effects of the Intermediate Fertility Variables," *Studies in Family Planning, 13,* 6/7, 179–189.

Henry, L. (1965), "French Statistical Research in Natural Fertility," in M. C. Sheps and J. C. Ridley, Eds., *Public Health and Population Change*, University of Pittsburgh Press, Pittsburgh, pp. 333–350.

Jones, E. F., L. Paul, and C. F. Westoff (1980), "Contraceptive Efficacy: The Significance of Method and Motive," *Studies in Family Planning, 11*, 2 (February), 39–50.

Laing, J. (1978), "Estimating the Effects of Contraceptive Use on Fertility," *Studies in Family Planning, 9*, 6 (June), 150.

McFalls, J. (1979), "Frustrated Fertility: A Population Paradox," *Population Bulletin, 34*, 2, Population Reference Bureau.

Menken, J., J. Trussell, K. Ford, and W. F. Pratt (1979), *Contraception: Science, Technology, and Application*, National Academy of Science, Washington.

Potter, R. G. (1971), "Inadequacy of a One Method Family Planning Program," *Studies in Family Planning, 2*, 1 (January), 1–6.

Potter, R. G. (1972), "Additional Births Averted When Abortion is Added to Contraception," *Studies in Family Planning, 3*, 4 April, 53–59.

Potter, R. G. and J. M. Sakoda (1966), "A Computer Model of Family Building Based on Expected Values," *Demography, 3*, 2, 450–461.

Potter, R. G. and J. M. Sakoda (1967), "Family Planning and Fecundity," *Population Studies 20* (March), 311–328.

Ryder, N. B. (1973), "Contraceptive Failures in the United States," *Family Planning Perspectives 5*, 3 (Summer), 133–142.

Sagi, P. C., R. G. Potter, and C. F. Westoff (1962), "Contraceptive Effectiveness as a Function of Desired Family Size," *Population Studies, 15* (March), 291–296.

Tietze, C. (1981), *Induced Abortion: A World Review, 1981*, 4th Ed., A Population Council Fact Book, The Population Council, New York.

Tietze, C. and J. Bongaarts (1975), "Fertility Rates and Abortion Rates: Simulations of Family Limitation," *Studies in Family Planning, 6*, 5 (May), 114–120.

Tietze, C. and S. Lewit (1973), "Recommended Procedures for the Statistical Evaluation of Intrauterine Contraception," *Studies in Family Planning 4*, 2 (February), 35–42.

Troen, P. and H. Oshima (1980), "The Male Factor," *The New England Journal of Medicine 303*, 13, 751–752.

Trussell, J. and J. Menken (1981), "Life Table Analysis of Contraceptive Use-Effectiveness," in Albert J. Hermalin and Barbara Entwisle, Eds., *The Role of Surveys in the Analysis of Family Planning Programmes*, Ordina Editions, Liege. pp. 537–571.

Vaughan, B., J. Trussell, J. Menken, and E. F. Jones (1977), "Contraceptive Failure Among Married Women in the United States, 1970–1973," *Family Planning Perspectives, 9*, 6 (November/December), 251–258.

Westoff, C. F. (1981), "Planned and Unplanned Births in the United States: 2. The Decline in Unwanted Fertility, 1971–1976," *Family Planning Perspectives, 13*, 2 (March/April), 70–72.

Westoff, C. F. and J. McCarthy (1979), "Sterilization in the United States," *Family Planning Perspectives, 11*, 3 (May/June), 147–152.

Westoff, C. F. and R. G. Potter, P. C. Sagi, and E. G. Mishler (1961), *Family Growth in Metropolitan America*, Princeton University Press, Princeton.

Westoff, C. F. and Norman B. Ryder (1977), *The Contraceptive Revolution*, Princeton, Princeton University Press.

8
Birth Spacing

INTRODUCTION

When family planning has reached an advanced stage in a society, most couples seek to control the timing as well as the number of their births. This chapter is concerned with the degree of spacing control attainable despite a variety of constraints, including fallible contraception, delays of conception once contraceptive precautions are suspended, and spontaneous pregnancy losses.

Several circumstances make an empirical analysis of birth-spacing control difficult, if not unfeasible. As will be documented later, most couples find it hard to articulate precise spacing goals. A broad range of birth-spacing experience may be adjudged retrospectively as acceptable. Subfertility or divorce may render spacing goals irrelevant. The two spouses may disagree about their spacing objectives. The two partners may be vague about their preferred birth intervals and inclined to put off discussion of the issue. For example, as suggested by Sagi, Potter, and Westoff (1962), a couple employing a coitus-related contraceptive, who are unable to make up their minds, can take occasional chances by omitting contraception precautions and, in effect, let fate determine the timing of their next pregnancy.

An attractive approach, made possible by appropriate reproductive models, is to investigate the limits of birth-spacing control under idealized conditions, namely, clear-cut, unchanging spacing goals in marriages that remain intact and free of natural sterility long enough for the couple to reach desired family size. Simulated each time is a hypothetical cohort of couples striving to realize a given common spacing goal and utilizing for that purpose a designated strategy respecting when to interrupt contraception. Actual timings of births vary stochastically among cohort members and their dispersion around intended birth schedules yields a measure of spacing control. The relevance of factors such as age at marriage, effectiveness of contraception, and nature of the spacing goal itself can be tested by varying their values in a series of simulation runs.

Two broad classes of spacing preference are usefully distinguished. First are master-schedule spacing preferences, already encountered in Chapter 7 and readily operationalized by REPMOD. Such intentions encompass as subgoals a preferred interval from marriage to first birth and a preferred childbearing span from first to last desired birth. The latter, together with the number of children desired, determines a preferred interval between consecutive births. Top priority is given to keeping as closely as possible to the implied birth schedule and by this means maximizing control over the timing of the last desired birth.

The second main class will be labeled "serial" spacing preferences. Here priority is given to having each birth interval of convenient length and accepting the childbearing span that results. A convenient length is one that does not fall short of a prefigured minimum or exceed a predesignated ceiling and ideally stays close to an intermediate, most preferred duration. It turns out that the representation of this type of spacing preference calls for a microsimulation model and is not feasible with REPMOD.[1] However, by accepting a few simplifying assumptions, the dynamics of controlling a single birth interval can be investigated by means of an analytical model, SPACE, designed for the purpose.

The rest of the chapter is organized by sections as follows. The previous literature on spacing attitudes is first reviewed as background for delineating in more detail master-schedule and serial-spacing preferences.

Examined second is the variability of the interval from marriage to last-desired child when contraception is not practiced. This variation, which reflects the cumulative chance effects of conceptive delays, spontaneous pregnancy losses, and postpartum anovulation, is shown to augment rapidly as the number of children wanted increases. It is this accumulation of chance variation across parity that must somehow be constrained if reasonably precise timing of the last birth is to be achieved.

---

[1] For REPMOD, the obstacle to simulating serial-spacing preferences is the need to keep track of the beginning dates of each birth interval. To translate a given month of marriage duration into an ordinal month with respect to the current birth interval requies knowing the marriage duration at which the birth interval started. Because of the wide range of these durations, the number of statuses to be kept separate becomes very large.

Next considered is the spacing control achieved in behalf of a master-schedule spacing preference by always interrupting contraception 1 year in advance of the intended date of the next birth unless that target is less than a year away, in which case contraception is waived altogether for that birth interval. It is demonstrated that couples willing to adjust subsequent birth intervals to compensate for any deviations from their master schedule encountered at early or middle stages of their family building secure sufficient control over the timing of their last-desired birth so that its variability increases only very slowly as the number of wanted children is enlarged. The qualifying effects on spacing control exercised by age at marriage, effectiveness of contraception, and width of preferred birth intervals are also studied.

Given a serial spacing goal, the aim becomes one of controlling the lengths of each of a succession of birth intervals. Once a most preferred date for the next birth is fixed, there arises the problem of when to interrupt contraception. Influencing this decision is the couple's perception of how long it will take to conceive once contraception is stopped. Four rules for predicting conceptive delays are specified and their efficiencies compared in the section titled "Serial Spacing." The main result of a rather complex analysis is that much more important than choice of estimation procedure is the level of the couple's natural fecundability. If the latter is low, all predictive rules lead to unsatisfactory results; when fecundability is high, the rules produce similar predictions and operate efficiently.

On the strength of this result, the issue of whether raising the rate of marital intercourse is an efficient means of elevating fecundability becomes a matter of considerable practical interest. It is shown, in the succeeding section, that given certain conditions, including freedom from subfecundity and the proper timing and duration of special efforts, that the strategy of heightened coital rates can prove remarkably effective in enhancing spacing control.

The last topic considered is the exploitation of high fecundability for purposes of "pinpoint spacing," that is, seeking to keep the next birth within a relatively brief period of 3 months or less. Here the proper strategy is to interrupt contraception at the start of the target period.

PREVIOUS STUDY

Though a large literature exists on birth intervals and their correlates, a much smaller literature pertains to spacing attitudes. This dearth of attention is not an accident. Couples find it difficult to articulate precise spacing goals.

Questions aked of mothers from the Princeton Fertility Study (Westoff Potter, Sagi and Mishler 1961), revealed that the two most salient considerations in respect to the best spacing between children are limiting the load of child care and assuring that the children become playmates. With regard to the latter issue, a birth interval exceeding 4 years is usually deemed too long; intervals under $2\frac{1}{2}$ years are typically regarded as safe; durations of $2\frac{1}{2}$–4 years leave room for argument. Less agreement prevailed concerning the manner in which spacing affects the exigencies of child care. A longer birth interval stretches out the period of intensive infant care, but a shorter birth interval increases the intensity of child-care responsibilities during the first few months after the second child arrives. The respondents exhibited a stronger consensus that if the first and second children are close in age, then the next birth interval should not be so short in order to avoid three small children in the house at once.

Among "relatively fecund" wives from the Indianapolis Study asked to describe the "most desirable" interval between first and second birth, altogether 86% said 2 years, 2 or 3 years, or 3 years (Whelpton and Kiser 1950). Mothers having two children from the Princeton Fertility Study were asked: "If you should decide to go on to a third child, how long from now would be the best time for it to be born?" Seventy-three percent reported a spacing ideal of 2–$3\frac{1}{2}$ years, with a substantial mode of 33% at 2.5 years (Westoff *et al.*, 1961). Thus, in both studies ideal intervals between children are usually set at 2 years up to $3\frac{1}{2}$ years.

Respondents from the Princeton Fertility Study, when all of them had recently had a second child, were also asked to rate the timing of their first born in terms of "too soon," "just right," or "too late." A wide range of grouped lengths, from 8 to 11 months up to 47–53 months, were accorded a majority of "all right" ratings, although only for lengths 18–23, 24–29, and 30–41 months were 75% or more of the responses "all right." A majority said "too late" to intervals of 54–71 months, whereas a majority professed the timing was too soon when the first birth came sooner than 8 months after marriage. Regarding the second interval between first and second births, over 85% judged intervals of 19–36 months just right. Even among wives experiencing second intervals of 13–18 or 37–48 months, majorities viewed them as just right (55% and 68%). As these statistics plainly show, couples have a hard time perceiving any narrow range of birth-interval length as peculiarly advantageous over other lengths.

In a later volume of the Princeton Fertility Study series, Bumpass and Westoff (1970) argued that birth intervals are primarily a function of desired family size. The more children wanted, the shorter birth intervals tend to be. They conclude that spacing preferences are more oriented to desired duration of child care than to specific lengths of given intervals.

The idealization of this priority, whose importance Bumpass and Westoff stressed, is embodied in what is being called "master-schedule" preferences. For purposes of simulation, these spacing goals have to be made more precise and more constant over time than they would be in real life. As simulated by REPMOD, they include a preferred interval from marriage to first birth and a preferred childbearing span from first to last birth, which, divided by the number of children desired, yields a preferred birth-to-birth interval. Together, the preferred intervals dictate a childbearing schedule. If the couple fall behind this schedule owing to slow conception or pregnancy losses, they try to catch up by a shorter next segment of contraception or, if necessary, by no contraception at all in the next birth interval. If they move ahead of schedule as the result of a contraceptive failure, they seek to lengthen appropriately their next segment of contraception. The crux is a willingness to sacrifice any postponement of the next pregnancy or to put up with a long contraceptive segment, if need be, in order to get back on schedule. Also built into the simulation of master-schedule preferences is a standard decision to interrupt contraception 12 months ahead of the time the next birth is wanted. As time to conception averages longer than 3 months, this decision rule carries a small bias in the direction of late births. An earlier study of master-schedule spacing preferences was conducted by means of another macrosimulation model, FERMOD (Potter and Sakoda, 1966, 1967) that lacks several of the refinements of REPMOD.

In the case of serial-spacing preferences, priority goes to having each birth interval command a reasonable length as dictated by current circumstances. Once the first child is born, there are four elements to consider in planning the next birth interval. There is a minimum length of birth interval to be insisted upon in order to limit the intensity of child-care responsibilities when the second child arrives; there is a ceiling length, relating to the playmate issue, not to be exceeded; and there is an intermediate, most preferred length. A fourth element is the decision rule guiding when to interrupt contraception in order to have the next birth as close to the target date C as possible. Three decision rules will be distinguished here. The relevance of any previous birth interval is its information on how quickly the couple conceived after suspending contraception.

UNREGULATED BIRTH SPACING

Useful background for the study of birth-spacing control under master-schedule preferences is what happens to the variability of timing of the last desired birth when no effort is made to control it by means of contraceptive practice. This variability of timing of a last desired birth of specified order will be measured by the standard deviation of marriage duration to that birth.

An important generalization is that variability of birth timing increases with birth order. Unconstrained by deliberate efforts at spacing control, chance effects accrete over parity. Other things being equal, variability is larger for the first birth and increases in absolute terms more rapidly with increasing birth order when postpartum anovulation is lengthy rather than brief. The same forecast holds when marriage takes place several years after rather than close to 20 years because, if marriage is started relatively late, childbearing is more likely to extend into ages characterized by nontrivial declines of fecundity. Of course, desired family size plays an important role as it sets the number of births over which chance variation in birth timing may accumulate.

These predictions are tested in Table 8.1, which, based on REPMOD runs, presents mean durations to last desired birth as well as corresponding standard deviations. When postpartum anovulation averages 3.0 months, chance effects depend almost entirely on the variabilities of conceptive delays and spontaneous pregnancy losses, whereas postpartum anovulation averaging 18.5 months adds a significant third source of chance variability. The two different regimens of postpartum anovulation occupy the top and bottom panels of Table 8.1. Desired family size defines columns so that by looking across rows one can see, for given marriage age and average length of postpartum anovulation, the increasing variability of duration to last wanted birth as desired number of children increases. Note that the standard deviations corresponding to fourth births are roughly 2.5 times larger than those characterizing first births. Stated otherwise, the variance of time of last wanted birth increases at a rate disproportionately faster than the number of children desired.

Three different marriage ages are compared in Table 8.1, the choices differing between long and short anovulation in order to represent age ranges into which a majority of first marriages might fall appropriate respectively to

Table 8.1

MEAN AND STANDARD DEVIATION OF DURATION FROM MARRIAGE TO LAST DESIRED BIRTH, GIVEN NO PRACTICE OF CONTRACEPTION, BY AGE OF WIFE AT MARRIAGE, MEAN LENGTH OF POSTPARTUM ANOVULATION, AND NUMBER OF CHILDREN DESIRED

Mean length of anovulation and marriage age	Number of children desired							
	1		2		3		4	
	Mean	SD	Mean	SD	Mean	SD	Mean	SD
Anovulation averages 3.0								
Marriage age:[b]								
20	16.57	8.60	36.11	13.08	55.68	17.15	75.30	21.13
25	16.65	8.76	36.40	13.57	56.30	18.30	76.48	23.11
30	17.40	10.15	38.55	16.41	59.98	21.65	80.80	25.05
Anovulation averages 18.5								
Marriage age:[b]								
16	22.77	13.34	59.71	21.48	96.04	28.17	132.3	34.23
20	17.92	10.19	54.27	19.85	90.71	27.09	127.0	33.48
25	18.02	10.39	54.70	20.70	91.68	28.52	127.3	33.22

[a] Length of anovulation and duration from marriage to last desired birth are measured in months.

[b] Measured in years.

"modern industrial" and "subsistence" conditions. Appreciable increases in the variability of birth timing, for a given desired family size, appears only for either very young marriage (for example, age 16) or else an advanced age (age 30, for instance).

MASTER-SCHEDULE SPACING

Master-schedule spacing preferences put emphasis on controlling the time of last desired birth. Two measures of spacing efficiency are applicable to couples who attain desired family size. First is the standard deviation of childbearing span, which commands the advantage of permitting comparisons between the situations of no-spacing control effort versus master-schedule spacing effort. A second measure is the proportion of couples succeeding in having their last wanted birth within a year of their target date. With respect to those who do not succeed, REPMOD distinguishes between those who are more than a year late or more than a year early.

Unless contraceptive effectiveness is perfect (i.e., $e_s = 1.0$), contraceptive failures occur and constitute an extra source of variability in addition to the stochastic variation of conceptive delays, spontaneous pregnancy wastage, and postpartum anovulation. Among wives wanting but one child, it can be anticipated that the standard deviation of intervals from marriage to that single birth will be larger when a postponement is attempted than when no effort at all is made to delay the birth, unless contraception is perfectly effective, in which case the standard deviation should be roughly the same in the two situations, as the factor of contraceptive failure as an extra source of variation is eliminated. However, as one passes to progressively larger desired family sizes over a range of one to four children say, the standard deviation of child-bearing span should increase much more slowly under a master-schedule spacing goal than in the absence of regulatory efforts.

It is evident that the effectiveness of contraception, e_s, plays a key role in both the proportion successful and the standard deviation of childbearing length. In any simulation of fertility subject to master-schedule spacing preferences, a crucial parameter is the value assigned to spacing effectiveness.

The most recent nation-wide data for the United States based on the concept of use effectiveness that permits classification by method and motive (delaying or preventing births) are the estimates, examined in Chapter 7, that were derived by Vaughan, Trussell, Menken and Jones (1977) from Cycle I of the National Survey of Family Growth. This study covers the 3-year period 7/1/70–7/1/73. The first column of Table 8.2, calculated as the complements of the 1-year failure rates taken from Table 7.9, shows that users of the different methods vary appreciably in the proportions who avoid accidental pregnancy for as long as a year. Corresponding estimates of effectiveness, e_s, are given in parentheses directly following the names of the method.

Table 8.2

**OBSERVED AND PROJECTED PROPORTIONS SUCCEEDING IN DELAYING
FIRST BORN AS LONG AS DESIRED, BY LENGTH OF INTENDED
POSTPONEMENT AND EFFECTIVENESS OF CONTRACEPTION, FOR WIVES
MARRIED AT 20 YEARS OF AGE**

Method of contraception [b/]	Intended delay of first pregnancy [a/] (years)				
	1 [c/]	2 [d/]	3	5	10
Pill (.991)	.980	.960	.941	.904	.817
IUD (.975)	.944	.891	.841	.750	.562
Condom (.935)	.863	.745	.643	.479	.229
Diaphragm (.924)	.841	.707	.595	.421	.177
Foam (.920)	.833	.694	.578	.401	.161
Rhythm (.852)	.712	.507	.361	.183	.033
All methods (.967)	.927	.859	.797	.686	.470

a/   Intended delay of k years signifies wanting the first birth at the end
     of the (k+1)th year of marriage.

b/   Values in parentheses represent estimates of contraceptive effective-
     ness derived from 12-month failure rates reported by Vaughan, Trussell,
     Menken and Jones (1977) for delayers.

c/   These 1-year success rates are calculated by taking complements of the
     1-year failure rates reported in the article by Vaughan, Trussell,
     Menken and Jones (1977).

d/   To convert a 1-year success rate into a k-year success rate, the
     former is raised to its kth power, based on the assumption that natural
     fecundability remains constant during ages 20-30.

Effectiveness exceeds .90 for all methods listed except rhythm. It equals
and exceeds .975 for IUD and the pill, respectively, and because of the
heavy weighting of these two methods stands at above .95 for all nonpermanent methods combined. Nevertheless, the proportions projected as escaping accidental pregnancy over specified numbers of years vary greatly among
the methods as the five columns of Table 8.2 demonstrate. Though about
80% of pill users might escape pregnancy over a decade, it is only slightly
above half of that for IUD wearers. The effectiveness levels of condom,
diaphragm, or jelly allow less than half of their practitioners to remain non-
gravid for as long as 5 years. For rhythm users, average effectiveness is low
enough to produce a 50% pregnancy rate in about 2 years.

The results of Table 8.2 are subject to two opposing biases. It is demonstrated by Trussell and Menken (1981) that among continuous practicers of
contraception, proportions surviving a year without accidental pregnancy is
higher during the second year of exposure than the first. From this
standpoint, the calculation underlying Table 8.2, that predicts chances of
surviving k years by raising the first-year survival rate to power k, is pes-
simistic. On the other hand, unplanned pregnancies during lapses of con-

traception are excluded. Substituting the concept of extended use-effectiveness for use effectiveness, Trussell and Menken (1981) lift the 1-year failure rate for all methods among delayers from .073 to .125.[2] Implied is an average effectiveness of .942, down from the .967 predicated upon continuous practice of contraception. A disproportionate number of the unplanned pregnancies during lapses of contraception are associated with the coitus-related methods inasmuch as continuation rates are materially lower for these methods than for the pill and the IUD.

Given such variation in spacing effectiveness, no one value can be construed as most typical for U.S. couples. In the REPMOD simulations to follow, spacing effectiveness is taken either as 1.0, to give an upper-bound estimate of spacing control, or as .90, to represent a low value corresponding roughly to, perhaps even slightly underestimating, the extended use-effectiveness of coitus-related contraceptives as employed by U.S. couples in the early seventies for purposes of delaying births.

For the simulations covered by Table 8.3, a modern context is assumed. Two marriage ages, 20 years and 30 years, are illustrated, and a range of desired family sizes from one to four children. As in Chapter 7, a *medium spacing goal* is defined as unpostponed first birth and 2 years sought between desired births, whereas a *wide-spacing goal* denotes seeking a 1-year extension of the interval to first birth and maintaining 3 years between consecutive children.

Consider first a marriage age of 20. If contraception is perfectly effective ($e_s = 1.0$), then there is no risk of attaining desired family size more than 12 months ahead of the target date. Under these conditions, a wide-spacing goal carries an advantage over a medium-spacing goal as it affords more opportunity to compensate for tardy intermediate births. As Table 8.3 shows, given a wide-spacing goal, the proportions P who keep their last desired birth within a year of their target date start at .88 when only a single child is wanted and decline only to .83 when four children are sought, signifying a high level of spacing control. The corresponding values for a medium-spacing goal are .87 and .76. In both instances, the standard deviation of duration to last desired birth increases with parity but much more slowly than in the absence of contraception, as a comparison with Table 8.1 demonstrates.

If spacing effectiveness is .90, then there exists a risk of completing childbearing more than a year ahead of schedule by virtue of one or more contraceptive failures. Moreover, the risk is higher for wide spacers who are seeking to maintain 3 years between children instead of the 2 years favored by medium spacers. Accordingly, when $e_s = .90$, a wide-spacing goal be-

---

[2] What Trussell and Menken report in Table 10 of their article are 1-year failure rates of .141 for black and .123 for white delayers. These two rates, weighted as .10 and .90 respectively, yield an overall .125. Conversion of this coefficient into effectiveness e_s is by Formula (4) of Chapter 3 with natural fecundability set at .19.

Table 8.3

STANDARD DEVIATION SD OF MARRIAGE DURATION TO LAST WANTED BIRTH AND PROPORTION P TIMING THAT LAST BIRTH WITHIN ONE YEAR OF TARGET DATE, BY NUMBER OF CHILDREN DESIRED, AGE OF WIFE AT MARRIAGE, EFFECTIVENESS OF CONTRACEPTION, AND MEDIUM OR WIDE SPACING GOAL[a]

Age at marriage, effectiveness, and spacing goal	Number of children desired							
	1		2		3		4	
	SD	P	SD	P	SD	P	SD	P
Wives marrying at age 20								
effectiveness $e_s=1.0$								
medium spacing a/	8.60	.87	11.02	.82	13.00	.79	14.94	.76
wide spacing	8.59	.88	9.67	.86	10.47	.85	12.04	.83
effectiveness $e_s=.90$								
medium spacing	8.60	.87	11.63	.82	13.76	.78	15.71	.76
wide spacing	9.65	.86	13.33	.72	15.74	.68	18.09	.65
Wives marrying at age 30								
effectiveness $e_s=1.0$								
medium spacing	10.15	.85	14.64	.76	18.17	.68	19.79	.62
wide spacing	10.79	.84	14.42	.76	16.30	.69	15.51	.64
effectiveness $e_s=.90$								
medium spacing	10.15	.85	15.13	.77	18.72	.69	20.30	.63
wide spacing	11.68	.83	17.14	.67	19.89	.61	19.64	.58

a/ See text for definitions of medium and wide-spacing goals.

comes disadvantageous and generates lower P values and higher standard deviations to last desired birth than a medium-spacing goal. In both instances, the rise of standard deviation as desired family size increases is more rapid than when $e_s = 1.0$, but less rapid than when contraception is absent.

Consider next a marriage age of 30. Here, because childbearing is extended into the middle or late thirties, the risk of spontaneous pregnancy wastage is enough higher and natural fecundability yet enough lower to impair spacing control over the last birth intervals. Furthermore, seeking 3 years instead of 2 years between births intensifies the problem. Nevertheless, when backed by contraception of perfect reliability, wide spacers preserve an advantage over medium spacers (at least when two or more children are sought) because of the greater opportunity to compensate for any tardy intermediate births. However, when spacing effectiveness is only .90, the advantage passes over to the medium spacers.

For any combination of spacing effectiveness and spacing goal, marriage at age 30 as compared to marriage at age 20 results in higher standard deviations of duration to last desired birth and proportions P keeping within 1 year of the target that decline more rapidly with an increase in the number of children wanted. These contrasts are made plain by comparing the last four rows of Table 8.3 with the first ones. Interestingly enough, given a marriage age of 30 and wide spacing, the standard duration of last birth-time, instead of rising progressively with larger desired family size, decreases between parity three and four, presumably as the result of a truncation effect.[3]

SERIAL-SPACING PREFERENCES

Serial-spacing preferences treat each birth interval in its own right. To simulate fertility under this kind of spacing goal, it is necessary to make spacing preferences more precise than would likely be the case in real life. Let us assume that the couple have had one child and can recall the length of the waiting time from interruption of contraception to first conception. With respect to the next birth, they want to avoid having it sooner than $\underline{m}$ months after the first birth. They have a most preferred birth interval length C. Finally they are anxious that the interval not exceed a ceiling length $\overline{m}$. Thus their spacing goal consists of a minimum interval $\underline{m}$, a target length C, and a ceiling duration $\overline{m}$. The challenge is to stop contracepting at a time that minimizes the expected deviation of second birth time from target date C.

The efficiency of a decision rule may be measured by the dispersion of birth times around the target date. For an individual couple, let the difference between actual and intended birth time be denoted as d. If the average of these differences in a cohort of couples following a decision rule is signified by $E(d)$ and the corresponding variance by σ_d^2, then the mean squared deviation is $E(d^2) = \sigma_d^2 + (E(d))^2$. When $E(d)$ deviates from 0, the decision rule is biased. The advantage of $E(d^2)$ as a measure of inefficiency over the variance σ_d^2 is that it is responsive to the "bias" $E(d)$ by virtue of the term $(E(d))^2$; whereas the variance is wholly insensitive to a failure to center second birth times on the target date.

Four decision rules merit comparison, two of the rules being naive, the

---

[3] Childbearing is extending into ages for which the proportion sterile rises rapidly. A truncation effect operates on the measured standard deviation of last desired birth-times by virtue of the fact that the later is a potential time of attaining desired family size relative to the target date the more likely it is to be obviated by secondary sterility and therefore not figure in the measured standard deviation at all. Note in Table 8.3 that this phenomenon gives rise to an exception of the rule that a lower P value associates with a higher standard deviation coefficient. Specifically, when marriage age is 30 and $e_s = .90$, the wide spacers have a lower proportion P within 1 year of the target date (.58 in comparison with .63) but notwithstanding have a lower standard deviation (19.64 as compared with 20.30). Presumably the wide spacers' relatively advanced ages of childbearing are simultaneously contributing to a lower proportion keeping within a year of the target date, but also a constrained standard deviation of last desired birth-times.

Another exception to the above rule is contributed by medium spacers married at age 30 who are practicing contraception of .90 and 1.00 effectiveness. As compared with the latter, the former experience more early attainments of desired family size and fewer late ones with opposite effects on the two coefficients P and standard deviation.

third based on linear regression being more statistically sophisticated, and the fourth a counsel of perfection as it requires that the couple kow their fecundability exactly. In the case of "A estimation", the couple define themselves as "average" and assume their next waiting time for conception after stopping contraception will be what is average for their population. Denote this average waiting time as $E(i)$. Regardless of the length of their previous conceptive delay, they intend to interrupt contraception $9 + E(i)$ months before the target date, that is, at the start of month C-9-$E(i)$. This rule is statistically naive for making no use of information about their previous conceptive delay.

The second rule is just as naive for grossly exaggerating the amount of information contained in the recalled interval to first conception. Under "R estimation" the couple assume that their next waiting time will repeat the previous one of length i, say. Therefore they interrupt contraception at C-9-i unless i is so large that C-9-i violates their minimum birth interval in which case they defer interruption until duration $\underline{m}$-9, the earliest time point that does not risk violating the minimum birth interval $\underline{m}$.

If a couple somehow know their fecundability $\hat{f}_n$ and if that natural fecundability may be viewed as essentially constant from month to month, then the expected length of their conceptive delay becomes $1/\hat{f}_n$. Accordingly an appropriate decision rule, identifiable as F estimation, is C-9-$1/\hat{f}_n$.

Finally, let us suppose that while the natural fecundabilities are known for the entire cohort of couples, the fecundabilities of individual couples are unknown and must be estimated from the known cohort distribution together with information about each couple's previous conceptive delay. In this situation, regression principles may be applied to derive a decision rule of the form C-9-α-βi. The parameters α and β allow for the fact that if the previous delay i is very short, it implies that the couple have higher fecundability than average for the cohort, but also may have had a conceptive delay shorter than might be expected from their unknown fecundability and, accordingly, their next conceptive delay probably will not be as short as the previous one. This more sophisticated decision rule weights more judiciously past experience than do the first two estimation principles described.

How may one derive values of $E(d)$ and $E(d^2)$ so as to be able to compare the efficiencies of the different decision rules? Ideally with a suitable microsimulation model, the careers of a cohort of couples could be followed in a detail comparable to that of REPMOD. A less expensive option is to allow a number of simplifying assumptions and so reduce the inquiry to a task that can be handled by an analytical reproductive model. Such a model, called SPACE, is reported in Potter and Kobrin (1981). Its assumptions, though not its algebra, is worth summarizing here. As it will turn out that the important factor is the couple's fecundability, not the decision rule they chose, it does no harm to exaggerate spacing control by assuming a number of facilitating conditions.

The simplifying assumptions are as follows:

1. The couple have had one planned birth and accurately recall the length of time they waited for conception after deliberately interrupting contraception.
2. Contraception practiced in behalf of timing the second birth is perfectly effective so that there is no risk of interrupting contraception earlier than intended.
3. The couple are spared intrauterine mortality; once conceiving a second time, a birth follows 9 months later.
4. They follow their chosen decision rule to the letter, be it interrupting contraception at $C\text{-}9\text{-}E(i)$, $C\text{-}9\text{-}i$, $C\text{-}9\text{-}\alpha\text{-}\beta i$, or $C\text{-}9\text{-}1/\hat{f}_n$.
5. Among couples fecundability is distributed according to a Beta-Type I distribution whose parameters, $a = 4.559$ and $b = 18.236$, yield a mean fecundability of .20 and a coefficient of variation of .41 (in keeping with a result cited in Chapter 6).
6. The natural fecundability of any individual couple remains constant during the second conceptive wait and has the same value as during the first conceptive wait.
7. By a straight forward argument,[4] assumptions 5 and 6 dictate the value of the two parameters of the regression decision rule ("E estimation"): $\alpha = 4.561$ and $\beta = .219$.
8. To simplify formulas further, the continuous Beta-Type I distribution of natural fecundabilities is replaced by a 9-point discrete distribution (point-values and weights are enumerated in Table 8.5). With this substitution, the mean conceptive wait for the population becomes $E(i) = 5.98$, very close to the mean implied by the continuous distribution, and the accompanying standard deviation is 7.11.

Note that several of the assumptions—perfect recall of the one previous conceptive delay, perfectly effective contraception, freedom from pregnancy wastage, constancy of fecundability across two birth intervals, and meticulous conformity to one's chosen decision rule—all operate to enhance, even to exaggerate spacing control.

Each simulation run of SPACE generates $E(d)$ and $E(d^2)$ values for a hypothetical cohort pursuing by means of a designated decision rule a given spacing goal defined by the parameters $\underline{m}$, C, and $\overline{m}$. Table 8.4 compares the

---

[4] The two parameters of this Beta Type-I distribution have values of $a = 4.559$ and $b = 18.236$. Suppose that this distribution of fecundabilities among couples remains fixed during $k + 1$ successive pregnancy intervals. Given that a particular couple has averaged $\overline{i}$ months in their past k waiting times, then the maximum likelihood estimate of their fecundability can be shown to be $\hat{f}_n = (a + k - 1)/(a + b + \overline{i}k - 2)$. Letting $k = 1$, so that ι becomes simply the previous waiting time i, and defining the couple's expected next waiting time $\hat{i}$ as $1/\hat{f}_n$, we have $\hat{i} = (a + b - 2 + i)/a = (a + b - 2)/a + i/a = \alpha + \beta i$. Substituting $a = 4.599$ and $b = 18.236$ gives $\alpha = 4.561$ and $\beta = .219$.

Table 8.4

MEAN DEVIATION E(d) AND MEAN SQUARED DEVIATION E(d²) OF BIRTH TIMES FROM TARGET DATE, BY ESTIMATION PRINCIPLE AND SPACING GOAL

Spacing goal	Principle of estimation a/							
	F		E		A		R	
	E(d)	E(d²)	E(d)	E(d²)	E(d)	E(d²)	E(d)	E(d²)
$\underline{m}$=12, C=18, $\overline{m}$=36	.98	48.20	.56	50.20	.00	50.52	2.22	55.94
$\underline{m}$=12, C=24, $\overline{m}$=48	.22	42.45	.14	48.66	.00	50.52	1.00	57.26
$\underline{m}$=12, C=24, $\overline{m}$=36	.22	42.45	.14	48.66	.00	50.52	1.00	57.26
$\underline{m}$=12, C=36, $\overline{m}$=48	.03	40.50	.11	48.46	.00	50.52	.30	66.04
$\underline{m}$=12, C=84, $\overline{m}$=96	.00	40.15	.11	48.39	.00	50.52	.00	77.44

a/ Estimation principle F stands for fecundability known; E for statistically efficient (regression) estimation; "A" for average fecundability assumed, and R for repeat of previous conceptive wait assumed.

four decision rules for five different spacing goals. The order from most to least efficient is fecundability known, regression, average fecundability assumed, and repeat of previous conceptive wait relied on. The important result is the narrowness of differences, especially among the first three cited. For all four decision rules, bias as measured by $E(d)$ is consistently small. The spread of efficiencies, measured by $E(d^2)$, is consistently modest among the fecundability known, regression, and average fecundability assumed estimators. The remaining decision rule predicated on repetition of a previous wait falls farther behind the others when the subinterval C-$\underline{m}$ is made long.

The four decision rules are so equal in efficiency because the really important factor turns out to be the couple's fecundability. When that is high, all four rules predict relatively short conceptive delays and are usually vindicated in those predictions and so perform very satisfactorily. Given low fecundability, a wide scatter of previous conceptive delays are experienced, which, except for the average fecundability decision rule, generates variable predictions for next delays. The actual next delays exhibit again a wide scatter whose lengths correlate only very weakly with the predicted values, the results being that all four decision rules perform unsatisfactorily.

This close dependence of efficiency on level of fecundability is illustrated in Table 8.5 which for spacing goal $\underline{m} = 12, C = 24$, and $\overline{m} = 36$ presents $E(d)$ and $E(d^2)$ values for each of the nine subcohorts making up the discrete population substituted for the Beta-Type I continuous one. For the highest few fecundabilities, biases are low and efficiency high, but on passing to lower and lower fecundabilities, biases $E(d)$ and inefficiencies $E(d^2)$ climb rapidly for all decision rules. Clearly, then, level of fecundability is the crucial factor; choice of decision rule a rather secondary factor.

Table 8.5
COHORT MEANS $E(d_j)$ AND MEAN SQUARED DEVIATIONS $E(d_j^2)$ OF BIRTH TIMES FROM TARGET DATE, BY ESTIMATION PRINCIPLES, GIVEN THE "STANDARD" GOAL OF $\underline{m}=12$, $C=24$, AND $\bar{m}=36$

Cohort fecunda- bility f_j	Cohort weight w_j	Cohort variance $(1-f_j)$ f_j^2	Principle of estimation [a]							
			F		E		A		R	
			$E(d_j)$	$E(d_j^2)$ [b]	$E(d_j)$	$E(d_j^2)$	$E(d_j)$	$E(d_j^2)$	$E(d_j)$	$E(d_j^2)$
.0170	.0002	3401.39	46.52	5593.50	48.57	5766.62	52.84	6198.78	47.88	5701.43
.0336	.0033	856.01	17.76	1171.43	20.72	1292.34	23.78	1421.57	19.75	1257.79
.0521	.0133	349.21	7.19	400.91	11.11	478.89	13.21	523.81	10.10	466.13
.0713	.0300	182.68	2.03	186.80	6.64	231.81	8.04	247.40	5.77	232.58
.0708	.0502	110.28	.00	110.28	4.13	131.25	5.03	135.61	3.51	139.73
.1538	.4456	35.77	.00	35.77	0.52	37.70	0.52	36.05	0.88	51.39
.2418	.3382	12.97	.00	12.97	-1.33	15.38	-1.84	16.37	0.15	22.50
.3349	.1034	5.93	.00	5.93	-2.23	11.20	-2.99	14.90	0.02	11.35
.4293	.0158	3.10	.00	3.10	-2.24	10.77	-3.65	16.43	0.00	6.13
$E(d)$ [c]			.22		0.14		.00		1.00	
$E(d^2)$ [d]				42.45		48.66		50.52		57.26

[a] See Table 8.4 for definition of these estimation principles.

[b] $E(d_j^2) = (1-f_j)/f_j^2 + [E(d_j)]^2$.

[c] $E(d) = \Sigma w_j E(d_j)$.

[d] $E(d^2) = \Sigma w_j E(d_j^2)$.

In sum, couples concerned with having a next conception close to a given date should not be overly concerned with elaborate formulas for predicting length of next conceptive delay; rather they should do their best to raise their natural fecundability to a high level because given such a level, they are well justified in simply stopping contraception a very few months in advance of their target date less 9 months. We now turn our attention to the topic of raising one's fecundability without specific medical assistance.

ELEVATING FECUNDABILITY

A more aggressive strategy of birth-spacing control than any considered thus far consists of deliberately raising one's rate of marital intercourse, estimating the elevated (natural) fecundability $\hat{f}_n$ thereby attained, and interrupting contraception at month $C - 9 - 1/\hat{f}_n$. Three problems must be solved. First is formulating a rule to convert coital rates into fecundabilities. Second is deciding when and how long during the intermenstrum are special efforts necessary in order to be confident of bracketing the brief fertile period. Third is using the length of the previous waiting time to check the presumption of reproductive normalcy. If that presumption must be rejected, then a more appropriate strategy is simply interrupting contraception at $\underline{m} - 9$. These three issues are considered in turn.

James (1979) has recently reviewed the evidence that coital frequency is the predominant determinant of natural fecundability. In an earlier study, Barrett and Marshall (1969) analyzed daily calendars carrying information on the timing of intercourse and ovulation, the latter estimated by basal body temperature (BBT), in a sample of 241 noncontracepting, British women of proven fertility. Their model predicts a rapid rise of fecundability with increasing coital frequency, from a fecundability of .14 for once-a-week intercourse up to a very high figure of .68 for daily intercourse. In a reanalysis of the same data, Schwartz, McDonald and Herchel (1980) find good agreement between their predictions and Barrett and Marshall's at low and intermediate coital rates but project an appreciably lower fecundability of .49 at a daily rate. The quite different derivation featured in Chapter 2, which assumes that the fertile period is about 2 days in length instead of several days, yields estimates of fecundability that are slightly lower than those of Schwartz *et al.*, starting at .13 for a once-a-week coital rate and reaching a plateau of .45 as daily rates of coitus are approached. Six fecundability estimates based on Formula (3) of Chapter 2 are given in the top row of Table 8.6.[5]

Each coital frequency, expressed as *coitions per week*, determines a

---

[5] So that parameter n may define integral frequencies of coitus per week, the second parameter M is taken as 7.0. Equation (3) becomes $f = .45 \{1 - (7 - n)(6 - n)/42\}$. Substituting either $n = 6$ or $n = 7$ yields $f = .45$.

Table 8.6

REQUIRED COITAL RATES FOR, AND EXPECTED OUTCOMES FROM, SEVERAL
AGGRESSIVE SPACING STRATEGIES

Expected outcome	Coitions per weeks					
	1	2	3	4	5	7
Fecundability f_n	0.13	0.24	0.32	0.39	0.43	0.45
Expected waiting time $1/f_n$	7.7	4.2	3.1	2.6	2.4	2.2
Interruption time	C-17	C-14	C-13	C-12	C-12	C-12
Mean squared deviation from C, $E(d^2)$ [a]	51.48	13.19	6.64	4.01	3.08	2.72
Critical waiting time for rejecting f_n hypothesis at:						
.05 level	21.51	10.92	7.77	6.06	5.33	5.01
.01 level [b]	33.07	16.78	11.94	9.32	8.19	7.70

[a] $E(d^2) = (1-f_n)/f_n^2$

[b] To reject the f_n hypothesis at the α level, the previous waiting time must must be at least $\ln\alpha/\ln(1-f_n)$.

fecundability $\hat{f}_n$. Predicted waiting times, $1/\hat{f}_n$, all of them less than 8 months, are given in the second row of Table 8.6, followed by the appropriate interruption times $C - 9 + 1/\hat{f}_n$ rounded to the next higher integer. Expected second-birth times resultant from the six strategies coincide with the target date because $C - m \geq 8$, implying no interruption times earlier than $m - 9$. With $E(d) = 0$ and the variance of waiting times $(1 - \hat{f}_n)/\hat{f}_n^2$ modest, the mean-squared deviations, $E(d^2)$, are impressively low, especially for those strategies predicated on coital frequencies of three times or more. Of course these impressive performances presuppose that the couple have assessed their elevated natural fecundability accurately, admittedly a feat difficult to achieve.

When in the menstrual cycle should special efforts commence and how long must they be sustained in order to realize the augmented fecundabilities f_n? Survey inquiry (Potter, Sagi and Westoff 1962) has shown that many U.S. couples are seriously misinformed about the positioning of the fertile period in the menstrual cycle. Efforts to hasten pregnancy are not likely to succeed unless the couple have realistic ideas about when to increase their sexual activity above customary levels. Even correct information about the physiology of reproduction is only part of the solution. The menstrual cycles of women typically vary appreciably with a strong positive skewness (Treloar,

Boynton, Behn and Brown 1967, Vollman 1977). The larger part of this variability and skewness is contributed by the preovulatory or follicular phase (Potter, Burch, and Matsumoto 1967). BBT charts, the most widely known and accessible ovulation dating technique, is practical mainly for telling that ovulation is past (Vollman 1977). If useful for indicating when to terminate special efforts, it is much less efficient for revealing when to start.

Calendars with daily records of the occurrence of intercourse kept by noncontracepting women and screened down to months of alleged isolated coitus, such as amassed by Vollman (1953), suggest that the probability of conceiving is virtually 0 before the eighth and after the twenty-third cycle day, a 2-week span. Much shorter spans of special effort, say during cycle days 11–16, or from Day −4 to +1 relative to predicted day of BBT shift, are likely to miss an appreciable fraction of fertile periods. Accordingly, for a near certainty of bracketing the fertile period, it is essential to sustain special efforts during a 2-week period, 1 week before and 1 week after the mid-period. From results given in Chapter 2, it would appear that the fertile period averages about 48 hr, and for that reason marital intercourse every other day should suffice to give a high likelihood of conception during an ovulatory cycle.

The fact that in the practice of artificial insemination by donor (AID), more and more reliance is being placed on inducing ovulation by such means as the 5-day administration of clomiphene citrate (Klay 1976) advertises the unsatisfactoriness of ovulation dating by the traditional methods of calendar rhythm, BBT, or observation of cervical mucus. Having AID patients keep a daily record of BBT and then timing one or two inseminations to occur shortly before the predicted time of temperature shift rarely produces a monthly rate of conception higher than .20, though complicating interpretation here is the varying strictness with which AID patients are screened for fecundity impairments.

A third issue is testing for reproductive normalcy. The length of previous waiting time is not very informative unless the couple retain some idea of their accompanying rate of marital intercourse. A waiting-time-to-conception of 1 year, despite a coital frequency of three or four times a week, would carry a strong presumption of subfecundity, whereas a 12-month waiting time predicated on an once-a-week rate of intercourse would afford inconclusive evidence of subfecundity.

What are the critical lengths of waiting time beyond which there is less than an .05 or .01 chance of fecundability being as high as $\hat{f}_n$, reckoned from estimated coital frequency during the previous interval? For estimated fecundabilities as high or higher than .39, these critical lengths fall below a year. For $\hat{f}_n = .13$, they considerably exceed 1 year. The relevant values are given in the bottom two rows of Table 8.6.

A previous waiting time long enough to justify rejecting the hypothesis of a fecundability as high as $\hat{f}_n$ leaves the couple with a choice between seeking medical assistance or relying on special coital efforts combined with inter-rupting contraception early. The latter choice would follow from the idea that the subfecundity condition does not remove the essential proportionality between coital frequency and fecundability, but only reduces the propor-tionality factor.

PINPOINT SPACING

In the service of a serial-spacing goal, the strategy to be followed, whether it involves an effort to raise fecundability or not, is properly aimed at reduc-ing the spread of birth times around the preferred date, and this objective is better realized, other factors being equal, if the average time of the next birth coincides with the target date. A special case of serial spacing is seeking to have the next childbirth occur within a brief period, for example, the month before, during, and after a target month C. Here, optimal strategy is to raise fecundability as high as possible and to interrupt contraception at start of month $C - 10$. In any large sample, exposed to the risk of conception, the highest monthly proportion conceives in the first month of exposure, the second highest in the second month, and so on. Among couples sharing a common fecundability f_n, the highest frequency of conceptions, namely f_n, occurs during the first month, $(1 - f_n)f_n$ during the second month, and $(1 - f_n)^2 f_n$ during the third month, or a total of $P(3) = 1 - (1 - f_n)^3$ during the 3 months. Values of $P(3)$ corresponding to the $\hat{f}_n$ values (.13, .24, .32, .39, .43, and .45) of Table 8.6 are .34, .56, .69, .77, .81, and .83, respectively. Accord-ing to these calculations, a fecundability of .24, corresponding to two coi-tions per week, suffices for a majority to conceive within 3 months. A high fecundability such as .39, dependent on four coitions per week, assures that over three-quarters conceive by the third month. The advantages of a high natural fecundability are manifest here too.

SUMMARY

This chapter focused on spacing control. In the absence of such efforts, the time of the last desired birth varies appreciably as the result of random variations from conceptive delays and numbers of spontaneous fetal losses. Lengthy annovulation adds still another source of variation. Moreover, this stochastic variation accumulates rapidly over successive births, meaning that the standard deviation of duration from marriage to last desired birth increases sharply as desired family size increases.

Two broad classes of spacing goal have been investigated. When pursuing a master-schedule spacing goal, the couple, trying to keep their successive births as close to their chosen schedule as possible, are always abbreviating or else prolonging their practice of contraception depending on whether they fall behind or forge ahead of their timetable and thereby gain a large measure of control over their childbearing span. The standard deviation of duration to last birth still increases as the number of children desired increases but the cumulation of variation is much slower than in the absence of spacing-control efforts. Highly efficient contraception largely removes the risk of attaining desired family size early. In a context of youthful marriage and efficient contraception, a wide- rather than a narrow-spacing goal favors spacing control by affording more opportunity to compensate for intermediate births that are late. However, the advantage switches from wide- to narrow-spacing goals if contraception is inefficient. When marriage is late, at age 30 say, a wide- as opposed to a narrow-spacing goal tends to push childbearing into more advanced ages when the risks of pregnancy wastage and decreased fecundability are heightened and control over the last birth interval is weakened.

Pursuing a serial-spacing goal, the couple takes each birth interval in its own right, which means a minimum and a maximum length that they do not wish to violate and a most preferred intermediate length that they aspire to. Optimum strategy is to raise natural fecundability as high as possible and then, unless subfecundity is suspected despite these efforts, to interrupt contraception shortly before 9 months prior to the target date for the next birth. A number of formal decision rules about when to interrupt contraception can be distinguished. However, when natural fecundability is low, none of these decision rules work very well, whereas if natural fecundability is high, all become efficient and lead to approximately the same prescriptions. An augmented rate of marital intercourse is effective in raising natural fecundability only if properly timed within the menstrual cycle and extended over a sufficient number of days to give a high probability of encompassing the fertile period. Any previous conceptive delays experienced by the couple should be exploited as a check on their reproductive normalcy inasmuch as a suspicion of subfecundity dictates suspending contraception early even if efforts to augment natural fecundability are being made.

If the quest is to initiate pregnancy within a brief span, such as a 3-month interval, then appropriate strategy is to stop contraception just before the start of the target period. Maximizing chances of conceiving within a brief interval calls for a somewhat different approach than seeking to minimize the dispersion of birth times around a target date.

REFERENCES

Barrett, J. C. (1971), "Fecundability and Coital Frequency," *Population Studies, 25* (July), 309–313.

Barrett, J. C. and J. Marshall (1969), "The Risk of Conception on Different Days of the Menstrual Cycle," *Population Studies, 23* (Nov.), 455–461.

Bumpass, Larry L. and C. F. Westoff (1970), *The Later Years of Childbearing*, Princeton University Press, Princeton.

Klay, L. J. (1976), "Clomiphene-Regulated Ovulation for Donor Artificial Insemination," *Fertility and Sterility, 27* (April), 383–388.

James, W. H. (1979), "The Causes of the Decline in Fecundability with Age," *Social Biology 26* (Winter), 59–73.

Potter, R. G., T. Burch, and S. Matsumoto (1967), "Long Cycles, Late Ovulation, and Calendar Rhythm," *International Journal of Fertility, 12* (Jan.–Mar.), 1, Part 2, 127–140.

Potter, R. G. and F. E. Kobrin (1981), "Active and Passive Principles of Birth Spacing Control," unpublished manuscript.

Potter, R. G. and M. P. Parker (1964), "Predicting the Time Required to Conceive," *Population Studies, 18* (July), 99–116.

Potter, R. G., P. C. Sagi and C. F. Westoff (1962), "Knowledge of the Ovulatory Cycle and Coital Frequency as Factors Affecting Conception and Contraception," *The Milbank Memorial Fund Quarterly, 40* (January), 46–58.

Potter, R. G. and J. M. Sakoda (1966), "A Computer Model of Family Building Based on Expected Values," *Demography, 3,* 3, 450–461.

Potter, R. G. and J. M. Sakoda (1967), "Family Planning and Fecundity," *Population Studies, 20* (March), 311–328.

Potter, R. G., J. M. Sakoda, and W. E. Feinberg (1968), "Variable Fecundability and the Timing of Births," *Eugenics Quarterly, 15* (September), 155–163.

Sagi, P. C., R. G. Potter, and C. F. Westoff (1962), "Contraceptive Effectiveness as a Function of Desired Family Size," *Population Studies, 15* (March), 291–296.

Schwartz, D., P. D. M. McDonald, and V. Herchel (1980), "Fecundability, Coital Frequency, and the Viability of Ova," *Population Studies, 34* (July), 397–400.

Treloar, A. E., R. E. Boynton, B. G. Behn, and B. W. Brown (1967), "Variation of the Human Menstrual Cycle through Reproductive Life," *International Journal of Fertility, 12* (Jan.–Mar.), 1, Part 2, 77–126.

Trussell, J. and J. Menken (1982), "Life Table Analysis of Contraceptive Use-effectiveness," in Albert J. Hermalin and Barbara Entwisle, Eds., *The Role of Surveys in the Analysis of Family Planning Programs*, Ordina Editions, Liege, pp. 537–571.

Vaughan, B., J. Trussell, J. Menken, and E. F. Jones (1977), "Contraceptive Failure Among Married Women in the United States, 1970–1973," *Family Planning Perspectives, 9,* 6, (November/December), 251–258.

Vollman, R. F. (1953), "Uber Fertilitat und Sterilitat der Frau innerhalb des Menstruations Cycles," *Archiv fur Gynakologie, 187,* 602–622.

Vollman, R. F. (1977), *The Menstrual Cycle*, Saunders, Philadelphia.

Westoff, Charles F., R. G. Potter and P. C. Sagi (1963), *The Third Child: A Study in the Prediction of Fertility*, Princeton University Press, Princeton.

Westoff, C. F., R. G. Potter, P. C. Sagi, and E. G. Mishler (1961), *Family Growth in Metropolitan America*, Princeton University Press, Princeton.

Westoff, C. F. and N. B. Ryder (1977), *The Contraceptive Revolution*, Princeton University Press, Princeton.

Whelpton, P. K. and C. V. Kiser (1950), "The Planning of Fertility," in P. K. Whelpton and C. V. Kiser, eds., *Social and Psychological Factors Affecting Fertility*, Vol. 2, Milbank Memorial Fund, New York, pp. 209–258.

9

Sex Preselection

INTRODUCTION

Sex preselection represents a potential extension of fertility control. Having investigated the regulation of family size in Chapter 7 and the control of birth spacing in Chapter 8, it is the object of the present chapter to consider the governing of sex composition and sequencing of children. Numerous studies have attested to the presence of sex preferences (Williamson 1976). It seems reasonable to suppose that in societies practicing extensive family limitation and birth spacing, many couples would be inclined to take advantage of techniques of sex preselection if they commanded some efficiency, were not too medically risky, and were widely available.

Rinehart (1975) distinguishes three classes of techniques. First is the manipulation of sperm in vitro in order to increase the proportion of Y-bearing sperm that will produce males, which, coupled with artificial insemination, becomes the means of elevating the probability of a boy. Second is altering conception probabilities by purposive timing of coitus or modification of the vaginal environment. A third approach is a midtrimester diagnosis of fetal sex followed by a selective abortion when necessary.

The first two sets of techniques aim at modifying the probabilities of conceiving a boy or girl. The main disadvantage of these techniques at present are their low efficiencies, isolated claims notwithstanding (Glass 1977; Reinhart 1975).

The third approach, based on amniocentesis and selective abortion, does not try to alter conception probabilities but only to eliminate those pregnancies fated to result in an unwanted outcome. Though this approach commands high efficiency, it carries the disadvantages of requiring diagnoses of fetal sex and potentially one or more midtrimester abortions with attendant birth delays.

The main objective of this chapter is to study the number of diagnoses and selective abortions and associated added pregnancies required to achieve specified family goals of four children or less by amniocentesis backed by selective abortion. The greater these numbers on average, the less attractive the technique, its efficacy notwithstanding. Then too, additional pregnancies means weakened birth-spacing control and, in extreme enough instances, heightened risks of subfertility through prolongation of the childbearing period.

An important distinction exists between two kinds of family goal. A "compositional goal" means that the couple want their children to conform to a specified sex composition (e.g., two boys and a girl) but are indifferent to the order in which sons and daughters arrive. Given a "sequential goal," they aim to control order (e.g., a boy, then a girl, and last the second boy) as well as composition. Sequential goals require that the sex of every birth be regulated. Compositional goals allow the couple to waive regulatory efforts until the outstanding children are all of one sex. A supplementary interest is, then, how different are the diagnostic and abortion loads associated with the two types of goal.

Just as important as expected values are the scatters around them. Even when the expected numbers of diagnoses and selective abortions averaged over couples are rather low, if the scatter around these averages is large enough so that a nontrivial minority of practitioners will by virtue of bad luck encounter heavy loads of diagnosis and abortion, the approach loses much of its appeal.

It is hardly feasible to study these issues of sex control by direct observation. One may anticipate that many, if not most mothers, on confronting one or two unfavorable diagnoses of fetal sex, would abandon their sequential or compositional goal and decide to accept the sex of the child they are carrying as all right. A proper simulation model, however, gives one full latitude. It allows one to create an indefinitely large cohort of hypothetical couples all willing and able to handle the stochastically varying loads of diagnostic and abortion thrust on them by their sex goal and strategy for assuring it. In this manner the full implications of a dogged, uncompromising pursuit of given compositional or sequential goals can be revealed.

Most previous simulation studies of sex preselection have related to the first two sets of techniques, or else have assumed no sex preselection technology at all. The main findings of these studies are covered in the next section. Surprisingly little attention has been accorded amniocentesis and selective abortion despite its exclusive claim to efficiency.

The chapter is organized as follows. After first reviewing previous simulation work, the main concepts and the assumptions of the analytical model to be used are next described. Its algebra, reported elsewhere (Kobrin and Potter, 1981), is not repeated. Results are presented in five sections. First examined are the means and variances of the numbers of pregnancies, diagnoses, and abortions associated with a single regulated birth. Second, by way of further background, probabilities of attaining sequential and compositional goals in the absence of any sex control technology are given. In the next two sections, the means and variances of pregnancies, diagnoses, and abortions connected with achieving the specified goals by means of amniocentesis and selective abortion are investigated. Finally, the consequences for spacing control of an insistence on sex control are looked at. The chapter ends in a summary that the general reader might prefer to turn to next.

PREVIOUS RESEARCH

Couples who deliberately interrupt their childbearing when a minimum number of sons, or a minimum number of daughters, or some combination of the two objectives are obtained, may be said to be following a "stopping rule." A practical question is whether stopping rules affect the sex ratio at birth, which is normally around 105 boys to 100 girls, equivalent to probabilities of $P_b = .512$ of a son and $P_g = .488$ of a daughter.

An essential part of the answer was provided by Weiler (1959) who proved algebraically that if couples do not differ in their probabilities P_b of producing boys and therefore are constant in their probabilities $P_g = 1 - P_b$ of producing girls, then stopping rules cannot alter the sex ratio at birth. On the other hand, if couples do vary appreciably in their propensity to have boys, stopping rules will influence the sex ratio. Moreover the direction of that effect is counterintuitive. For instance, if a set of couples are following the stopping rule of no more children after the second son is born, the effect is to lower, not raise the sex ratio. This result follows because couples predisposed to have daughters will have to bear more children on the average in order to bear two sons than will couples predisposed to have boys. The lower-then-average sex ratio of the children of the former therefore receives more weight in the overall sex ratio than the higher-than-average sex ratio of the latter. Weiler's article corrected an earlier one by Winston (1932) who had come to the more commonsensical, but fallacious conclusion that the sex ratio would be raised.

Goodman (1961) distinguishes three different stopping rules directed to sons only, a balance of the two sexes, and a mixed preference (namely one daughter if she is the first born but otherwise at least one child of each sex), and then proceeds to derive general formulas for the sex ratio in each of the three cases contingent on the propensity P_b for sons varying among couples in a known manner.

This theoretical work has lent interest to the empirical question of whether heterogeneity with respect to P_b exists among couples. James (1975) concludes that boy propensity tends to decline with advancing parity, in part, because of an association with declining coital frequency. At the same time a variation of boy propensity exists among couples, this variation being demonstrated by the weakly contrasting sex compositions of next births among couples classified by sex composition of previous children. James notes that Malinvaud (1955) has reduced the dependence between the genders of past and present childbearing to the following linear relationship:

$$p_i = 51.45 + 0.3n_i - 0.5m_i.$$

Here p_i is the probability estimate, measured as a percentage, that the next pregnancy of the ith couple will yield a boy, n_i being their number of previous sons and m_i the number of their previous daughters. Malinvaud's regression suggests that heterogeneity with respect to son propensity is not large and may be ignored in simulation work without fear of major distortion, a simplification exploited in the main analysis of this chapter.

It has been already seen in Chapter 7 that, without a sex preselection technology, couples seeking two or three sons need a variably larger number of children to encompass the variable numbers of daughters they will have before the last desired son. Generalizing the issue slightly, one may ask how many children are necessary to have a minimum of b boys and g girls. Excluding multiple births, the minimum number of confinements is $b + g = N$, but may be appreciably larger. Table 9.1 presents the probabilities of requiring 0, 1, 2, . . . up to 5 or more additional births and their mean number, for all possible goals in the range of $N = 1$ to $N = 4$. These results are extracted from an analysis by Sheps (1963) in which it is assumed that the probability P_b of a boy is .515 and that of a girl, P_g, is .485.[1]

As one might expect, the probability of not requiring a single extra birth (first column of Table 9.1) declines as the minimum numbers wanted $b + g = N$ increases and, for fixed N, decreases as b and g are made more dissimilar. For example, there is only a 37% chance of achieving a balance of two boys and two girls in a four-child family, but a 50% chance of having one of each sex in a two-child family. At the same time, if family size is restricted to two

---

[1] In one of her two tables, Sheps considers mean family sizes when b boys and g girls are wanted and either no upper limit is imposed on childbearing or else an upper limit of k children, $k \geq b + g$, is set. Another table offers cumulative probabilities of realizing b boys and g girls within $b + g + h$ births. First differences of these values yields the probabilities of attaining the family goal in exactly $b + g + h$ births, reported in Table 9.1.

Table 9.1
PROBABILITIES OF REQUIRING SPECIFIED NUMBERS OF EXTRA BIRTHS AND
THEIR MEAN WHEN SEEKING A MINIMUM OF B BOYS AND G GIRLS, THE
PROBABILITY OF A BOY BEING .515

| Minimum Number | | | Extra births required | | | | | | Mean extra births |
Boys (b)	Girls (g)	Total (n)	0	1	2	3	4	5 or more	
1	0	1	.515	.250	.121	.059	.028	.027	.94
0	1	1	.485	.250	.128	.067	.034	.036	1.06
2	0	2	.265	.257	.188	.120	.074	.096	1.88
0	2	2	.235	.243	.187	.128	.087	.120	2.12
1	1	2	.500	.249	.125	.063	.031	.032	1.00
3	0	3	.137	.195	.193	.156	.113	.206	2.83
0	3	3	.114	.176	.182	.156	.120	.252	3.19
2	1	3	.386	.253	.151	.091	.052	.067	1.38
1	2	3	.363	.246	.157	.097	.060	.077	1.58
4	0	4	.070	.137	.165	.161	.136	.331	3.78
0	4	4	.055	.110	.147	.151	.137	.400	4.25
3	1	4	.265	.227	.173	.123	.081	.131	2.11
1	3	4	.235	.221	.170	.120	.080	.174	2.41
2	2	4	.374	.250	.156	.094	.055	.071	1.51

children, the goal of one son and one daughter will be reached roughly twice as often as the single-sex goals of two boys or two girls. Given family sizes of four children single-sex objectives of four sons or four daughters are more than five times as difficult to attain without extra births as a balanced preference of two boys and two girls, whereas the probabilities of attaining the partially unbalanced goals of three sons and a daughter or else three daughters and a son within four births are intermediate in value.

Inspection of Table 9.1 indicates that the higher the mean number of extra births required to achieve the compositional goal (last column of table), the greater the variability in number of extra births (intermediate columns) and the lower the probability of reaching the goal without any extra births (first column of table). It may be noted that attaining a single-sex goal involving two children ($b = 2, g = 0$ or $b = 0, g = 2$) occasions higher mean numbers of extra births and more variation among couples than does a balanced goal ($b = g = 2$) of four children. Thus, symmetry of compositional goal is as important as the total children desired.

If one subtotals coefficients across rows in Table 9-1, one obtains the cumulative probabilities of attaining the minimum quotas b and g of sons and daughters within designated sizes of sibships, the figures which Sheps (1963) reports. For some compositional goals, especially the larger, less-balanced objectives, these cumulative probabilities increase slowly. For these cases, one knows that many couples would abandon their compositional goal after one or two additional births. Family size considerations are paramount enough relative to gender interests so that unless the latter can be realized within 0, 1, or 2 extra births, they will be forfeited for the sake of a ceiling on total childbearing. From this standpoint, Table 9.1 offers a very hypothetical result, namely, the distributions of extra births that couples would have if particular compositional aspirations were so important to them that they stubbornly persist in, and have the physiological capacity for, continuing to childbear until the predesignated minimums b and g are both satisfied.

Suppose that by some set of sex preselection techniques the conditional probabilities P_b of having a boy when a son is wanted and P_g of having a girl when a daughter is wanted have been significantly elevated above their normal values of .512 and .488. In the special and rather hypothetical case of $P_b = P_g$, we speak of an "unbiased technology" whose efficiency is measured by the difference $P_b - .512$.

McDonald (1973), with extensions of his algebra by Smith (1974), has considered the problem of optimum strategy given an unbiased technology in the sense just defined. At each pregnancy there is a decision to be made whether to raise chances of a son up to P_b, chances of a daughter to P_g, or let nature "decide." A strategy consists of specifying in advance just what choices will be made at each pregnancy given the sex composition preferred together with the various gender outcomes of previous births. That strategy which maximizes chances of attaining the compositional goal in $b + g$ births is defined as optimal. McDonald also defines what he calls the "symmetry decision rule." If at any stage more boys are wanted than girls, raise to P_b chances that the next child will be a boy; if at any stage more girls are wanted than boys, raise to P_g chances that the next child will be a daughter; if the number of outstanding sons and daughters agree, let nature decide. In his main illustration, McDonald postulates $P_b = .885$ and $P_g = .864$, taken from the claims of Rorvik and Shettles (1970).

Under optimum strategy, the mean number of births required to achieve a compositional goal of b boys and g girls are drastically reduced from values predicated on no sex preselection technology. Unfortunately, the degree of sex control claimed by Shettles now appears as grossly exaggerated (Glass 1977 and Rinehart 1975). It turns out that with the probabilities adopted by McDonald (i.e., $P_b = .885$ and $P_g = .864$) the symmetry rule yields results closely approximating those of the optimal strategy. For example, under optimal strategy, mean number of births to achieve at least two boys and two girls is 4.15, whereas under the symmetry rule it is 4.163, a trivial difference. However, as the sex preselection technology becomes more biased, the symmetry decision rule tends to diverge from the optimal one at least for two-sex compositional goals.

McDonald also demonstrates marked sex-ratio effects. This result is illustrated by the compositional goal of one son or one daughter. In the former case, the expected ratio of sons to daughters is .885 to .115; in the latter case, it drops to .136 to .864. The more asymmetrical the compositional goal, the more extreme is the average sex ratio generated. Then too, even more extreme sex ratios for asymmetrical goals would have been predicted had values of P_b and P_g closer to 1.0 been posited.[2]

As different technologies are likely to be involved in raising the conditional probabilities P_b and P_g, the more general and realistic case is that which treats P_b and P_g as possibly unequal. For instance, procedures for partially separating out Y-bearing sperm may enhance P_b but leave P_g unaffected. To illustrate a biased technology, Mason and Bennett (1977) consider optimum strategy predicated on $P_b = .90$ and $P_g = .50$.

Their definition of an optimum strategy is one which maximizes the probability of achieving the compositional goal within $b + g$ births. Here a principle more useful than the symmetry decision rule is always to try for the "harder" sex, that is, in the present instance, for a daughter as the conditional probability P_g is so much lower than its counterpart P_b, unless the outstanding children wanted are all or predominantly boys. How extreme the predominance of boys must be before switching to an attempt to make the next child a son cannot be formulated in general, but must be derived by a computer calculation. Moreover, switching criteria in behalf of a given compositional goal may vary with differing values for, and degrees of inequality of, P_b and P_g.

The two authors provide a table of maximum probabilities of acquiring S additional sons out of C additional births with an accompanying indication of which immediate objective, a son or daughter, is preferred strategy. Thus at each stage of family building from consideration of the first birth to the $(b + g)$th, the couple, knowing the numbers of sons and daughters still outstanding, can by reference to the table aforementioned, determine the target for the next pregnancy. Not surprisingly, because the posited P_b so far exceeds the posited P_g, a goal of C children favoring sons is easier to achieve than one favoring daughters. Unfortunately, a different table has to be prepared for each postulated pair of P_b and P_g values. Mason and Bennett also consider the effects of optimum strategies upon the sex ratio.

AN ALTERNATIVE APPROACH

The development of amniocentesis as a means to predict and prevent through abortion the birth of infants with genetically determined birth defects has made possible selection on another genetically determined characteristic—gender. As the most frequently tested-for condition, Down's

---

[2] An interesting additional point made by Smith (1974), and illustrated with reference to the goal of two boys and one girl, is that the strategy which maximizes the probability of attaining the goal within $b + g$ births does not always minimize the expected number of births to attainment of the goal. This lack of synchrony somewhat dilutes the concept of optimal strategy.

syndrome, is associated with an inappropriate number of sex chromosomes, and as many other genetic abnormalities, such as hemophilia, are sex linked, a major concern in the development of amniocentesis techniques has been the accurate prediction of fetal sex. The technique used, karyotypic analysis of cultivated amniotic fluid cells, has been shown in a recent study to predict infant sex successfully in 99.93% of the cases. There were only two karyotyping errors in a group of 3000 amniocenteses (Golbus, Longham, Epstein, Halbasch, Stevens and Hall 1979). This contrasts sharply with the inefficiency of other approaches to sex preselection that have been developed so far (Glass 1977; Rinehart 1975).

Given that abortion is relatively unrestricted through the end of the second trimester, and as the results of amniocentesis can be known during this trimester, there now exists an essentially infallible means for realizing one's preferred sex composition. However this neigh perfect efficiency comes at a price: The numbers of diagnoses and abortions required can be substantial. Both the diagnoses and the corrective, midtrimester abortions entail medical risks. Furthermore, when additional pregnancies are required, they may lead to awkwardly prolonged birth intervals. Control over sex composition tends to compromise control over birth spacing.

Much of the debate concerning amniocentesis and selective abortion as a means of sex preselection has focused on the ethical and medical aspects. The purpose of the calculations presented in the rest of this chapter is simply to estimate how many of these procedures would be required to achieve a sex-tailored family and to note the consequences for birth spacing.

Two kinds of family goal will be considered. Under a compositional goal, the couple aspire only to control the sex composition of their children; if actuated by a sequential goal, they seek to control the sequencing of their sons and daughters as well. It will be shown how much less taxing is the realization of a balanced compositional goal such as two sons and two daughters as compared to achieving any of the associated sequential goals. None of the simulations reviewed in the previous section of this chapter treated sequential goals involving both boys and girls.

Nor did any of these previous simulation studies of sex preselection give explicit attention to spontaneous fetal wastage. Yet it is important to do so even if the algebra is thereby made more complicated because these involuntary fetal losses contribute to the number of pregnancies occurring within a birth interval, which, in turn, curtails the precision of birth spacing.

Using a small set of simplifying assumptions, a series of algebraic relationships may be derived. This algebra, taken from Kobrin and Potter (1981), rests on the concept of a "birth trial." A *birth trial* is a process that begins with the first pregnancy of a birth interval and ends with the birth that closes the interval. An unregulated birth trial, in which nature is allowed to "decide" the sex of the child, may encompass more than one pregnancy as the result of spontaneous pregnancy wastage. A regulated birth trial embraces one or more diagnoses of fetal sex and, contingent on their verdicts, possibly one or more corrective abortions, in addition to any pregnancies associated with spontaneous fetal losses.

As amniocenteses and any ensuing corrective abortions are performed during the second trimester, most spontaneous pregnancy losses will occur before these events, a small minority afterward. We will refer to those spontaneous abortions that occur before the time of a selective abortion as "early" and the rest as "late." Taking θ_2 as the total risk of spontaneous pregnancy loss, we denote θ_2^* as the proportion of "late" spontaneous abortions and $\theta_2 - \theta_2^*$ as the proportion of "early" spontaneous abortions.

Goals requiring a determination of fetal sex for each birth are the most costly in terms of the number of diagnoses expected (*diagnostic load*) and the number of abortions as well (*abortion load*). This will be the case for any sequential goal, as well as compositional goals involving only one sex. Other compositional goals make possible the development of an abortion-reducing strategy, or decision rule, that allows birth trials to proceed without regulation until the residual composition (the desired sex composition of the children yet unborn) includes only children of one sex. For example, if the family goal is two boys and two girls, at least two birth trials can go unregulated if either two boys or two girls are born, leaving a residual composition either of two girls or two boys, and can go to three trials if the first two births result in either sequence of a boy and a girl, so that the residual composition still includes a child of each sex. The last birth trial, however, will always be regulated. Under the abortion-reducing strategy, then, the number of unregulated birth trials is a random variable depending on the sex composition desired and the gender outcomes of the initial births.

ASSUMPTIONS

Six assumptions underlie this analysis:

1. Each diagnosis is interpretable and perfectly reliable.
2. Risks of "early" and "late" spontaneous abortion are constant among women and over the birth trials of individual women. Given that selective abortions are done at Week 20, these risks are $\theta_2 - \theta_2^* = .15$ and $\theta_2^* = .02$. respectively.
3. The fetal sex ratio at time of diagnosis equals 105, identical to the sex ratio at birth. This is equivalent to male and female proportions of .512 and .488.
4. Plural births are insignificant in number.
5. Family goals remain fixed, and couples attempt to realize them independently of the results of intermediate outcomes.

6. Couples are able to have as many pregnancies as are demanded by the conjunction of their family goal, chosen decision rule, and diagnostic outcomes.

The first three assumptions are approximately true, and whereas the fourth, on plural births, is not, it causes little distortion in exchange for great algebraic simplification. The last two are much more problematic, but underlie the central question of analysis.

With regard to the first assumption, it is true that a repeat amniocentesis is sometimes necessary because of failure to obtain clear, cell-bearing amniotic fluid or subsequent laboratory failure. However, Golbus et al. (1979) reported successful culture in 98.3% of the cases on the first attempt, and 99.7% when second attempts were included. Given successful culturing, their karyotypic diagnoses were essentially 100% reliable.

Respecting the second assumption, risk of spontaneous abortion varies markedly by age of women. In keeping with estimates cited in Chapter 2, the average risk level during ages 20 to 40 years is taken as .17. When this value is substituted into Nortman's age function, the estimated risk of pregnancy loss reaches its lowest value of .11 or .12 for women in their early twenties and climbs to a value around .30 for women in their very late thirties.[3] Unavoidable delays typically mean that any corrective abortions take place 2 and, more likely, 3 or 4 weeks after amniocentesis. In the algebra employed, this separation in time is ignored and the two events, amniocentesis and selective abortion, are assumed to occur simultaneously at Week 20.[4] Accordingly, the risk of late abortion, rounded to two decimal places, is set at $\theta_2^* = .02$, an estimate taken from the gestational age schedule given in Chapter 2. Implied is an incidence of early abortion of $\theta_2 - \theta_2^* = .15$. Although it has been generally anticipated that amniocentesis would increase the probability of late fetal loss, a number of studies to date have reported loss rates after amniocentesis that are not noticeably elevated relative to French and Bierman's results in the absence of such a procedure (cited in Golbus 1979).

---

[3] Nortman (1974) estimates the risk of spontaneous fetal loss as a function of age X (in years) by

$$R(X) = (.805 + .004 (X - 21.4)^2) .84C,$$

C signifying the average level of $R(X)$ over ages 20–40. Given $C = .17$, $R(21) \doteq R(22) \doteq .115$, a minimum value; whereas $R(39) = .292$ and $R(40) = .312$, almost three times as high.

[4] Treating the two events as simultaneous greatly simplifies formulas. Being ignored is the small incidence of spontaneous abortions that by occurring during weeks 16–19 do not forestall a diagnosis of fetal sex, but may obviate a corrective abortion. By referring diagnoses to the later gestational age, Week 20 instead of Week 16, their number is slightly underestimated, the error however being less than 1%. Based on the gestational age schedule of Chapter 2, out of 100 initiated pregnancies, an average of 82.1 diagnoses could happen if they were timed for Week 16 and 81.5 if the timing was Week 20. Thus the error involved in the 1-month displacement, namely the complement of .815/.821, is less than .01.

The third assumption, regarding the fetal sex ratio, relies primarily on the work of Yamamoto, Ito and Watanabe (1977). Sex was determined on aborted fetuses, and the sex ratio was found not to vary in any substantial way by length of gestation. This assumption also implies that the probability of conceiving a child of a given sex is independent of parity and previous outcomes. This would not be true if for some reason couples were heterogeneous with regard to expected sex ratios. Then families whose first child is a given sex would be selective of those prone to having that sex, and less likely to include those prone to having the other sex. James (1975) argues that such heterogeneity exists arising from variation in coital frequency, but the effect seems to be very small.

The final two assumptions are problematic, but necessary to allow the analysis to proceed. We are asking, essentially, "What will happen if family goals remain fixed, in the face of the diagnostic and abortion loads expected?" Therefore, family goals cannot be rationalized to fit the outcomes of intermediate pregnancies, nor can an unfavorable diagnosis be reacted to by deciding that the sex of the child being carried would be alright, after all. In effect, the fifth assumption means that these are the results that would obtain for those whose family compositional goals would not be altered in any way. If Assumption 5 implies that couples are willing to proceed as originally planned, no matter what, Assumption 6 requires that they be able. No allowance is made for the progress of secondary sterility as pregnancies mount. This assumption assures, along with Assumption 1, a 100% probability of attaining the family goal.

BIRTH-TRIAL PROBABILITIES

For unregulated birth trials, the number of diagnoses and selective abortions will be 0, and the number of pregnancies does not depend on the sex of the child. The only factor influencing that number in an unregulated birth trial is spontaneous abortion. Given a constant risk of spontaneous abortion over all pregnancies of $\theta_2 = .17$, the probability that a birth will require a given number of pregnancies looks like this:

Number of pregnancies	Probability
1	.830
2	.141
3	.024
4 or more	.005

Five-sixths need only one pregnancy to produce a birth; about one-seventh require exactly two pregnancies; and an unlucky 3% will need three or more. The average is $(1 - \theta_2)^{-1} = 1.20$ pregnancies, with a variance of .25 pregnancies per unregulated birth trial.

Introducing a sex constraint, however, raises the number of pregnancies required to achieve a child of a given sex substantially. Table 9.2 indicates that the number of pregnancies per regulated birth trial is 2.35 where a son is concerned, and 2.47 for a daughter. This reflects roughly a 50% chance of an unfavorable diagnosis each time one is performed, and a .15 chance of a spontaneous abortion before a diagnosis can be performed. The pregnancy variances are appreciable, their square roots being slightly more than three-quarters of the mean. Although nearly half of those successfully carrying a child of the desired sex would require only one diagnosis and no corrective abortion, the skewed distribution results in an average number of diagnoses of roughly two per birth trial, and corrective abortions of 1.0. Favorable diagnoses do not exactly equal 1.0 because of the small risk, namely .024, that a pregnancy associated with a favorable diagnosis will end in late spontaneous abortion or stillbirth.

When a daughter rather than a son is desired, the probability of an unfavorable diagnosis is slightly higher, .512 compared to .488, so that expected pregnancies, diagnoses, and corrective abortions are slightly higher when a daughter is desired compared to a son.

Notice has already been taken of the dependence of spontaneous abortion risk on age of the mother. The main effect of a higher or lower spontaneous abortion risk θ_2 is to raise or lower the expected number of pregnancies per birth trial. As this principal effect has a bearing on spacing control, discussion of the role of age is best reserved for that section of this chapter relating to spacing control.

Table 9.2

MEANS AND VARIANCES OF PREGNANCIES, DIAGNOSES, AND CORRECTIVE ABORTIONS IN A REGULATED BIRTH TRIAL, BY SEX OF CHILD DESIRED[a]

Event	Son desired		Daughter desired	
	Mean	Variance	Mean	Variance
Pregnancy	2.35	3.18	2.47	3.63
Diagnosis	2.00	2.01	2.10	2.31
Favorable diagnosis	1.02	.02	1.02	.02
Corrective abortion	.98	1.93	1.07	2.23

[a] Table A-1 in Kobrin and Potter (1981) for formulas. Parameter assignments are $\theta_2 = .17$, $\theta^*_2 = .02$; and the probability of a favorable diagnosis, $h = .512$ or .488, depending on whether a son or daughter is desired.

Table 9.3

PROBABILITY OF ACHIEVING A SEQUENTIAL OR COMPOSITIONAL FAMILY
GOAL IN THE ABSENCE OF SEX PRESELECTION TECHNOLOGY AS A
FUNCTION OF TOTAL BOYS AND GIRLS WANTED[a]

Number of boys b and girls g wanted	Any sequential goal	Compositional goal	Difference in probability
b	.512	.512	.000
g	.488	.488	.000
bb	.262	.262	.000
bg	.250	.500	.250
gg	.238	.238	.000
bbb	.134	.134	.000
bbg	.128	.384	.256
bgg	.122	.366	.244
ggg	.116	.116	.000
bbbb	.069	.069	.000
bbbg	.065	.262	.197
bbgg	.062	.375	.313
bggg	.060	.238	.178
gggg	.057	.057	.000

[a] The probability of achieving a sequential goal involving b boys and g girls is $(.512)^b (.488)^g$; that of the corresponding compositional goal is $\binom{b+g}{b}(.512)^b (.488)^g$.

A higher or lower risk of spontaneous abortion has little effect on either the expected diagnostic or selective abortion loads.[5] Accordingly, for most of the analysis, the level of spontaneous abortion risk θ_2 may be kept fixed at .17.

FAMILY COMPOSITION WITHOUT SEX PRESELECTION

Let us next consider what the absence of a sex selection technology means with respect to probabilities of achieving specified compositional and sequential goals. Table 9.3 presents these probabilities for all possible goals involving four children or less. In general, a compositional goal is easier to achieve than a sequential goal, except in the case where the composition involves only one sex, in which case sequence is in fact fixed, as well. As

[5] As the rate of spontaneous abortion ranges from .11 to .30, the expected number of diagnoses per regulated birth trial aimed at a male child varies only from 2.00 to 2.01. The corresponding change for the expected number of corrective abortions is only .97 to .98.

size increases, and as the preferred sex ratio is more unbalanced, the chances of achieving a given composition fall, and compositions emphasizing girls are more difficult to achieve than those featuring boys. For example, the easiest compositional goal to achieve involving three children, which is any sequence of two boys and a girl, can be expected with a probability of .384. This is a more likely outcome than any four-child composition or any other three-child composition.

For sequential goals, size again reduces the probability of a given outcome, and even more rapidly than for compositional goals. Sex balance is not a favorable factor; rather, for a given size, the more boys desired the greater the chances the goal will be realized. As a result, the difference between sequential goals and compositional goals increases the larger is the number of children wanted or, for a given family size, the more balanced is the goal.

These relationships parallel those which appear in the next two sections governing the number of pregnancies, diagnoses, and selective abortions required using selective abortion to achieve a given family size goal. The more difficult a goal is to achieve, the more pregnancies, diagnoses, and abortions that are required.

SEQUENTIAL GOALS

The most demanding of the family goals in terms of diagnostic and abortion loads and total pregnancies are the sequential family goals. These require that all $k = b + g$ birth trials be regulated. The expected numbers of pregnancies, diagnoses, and abortions as well as their variances depend on the numbers of girls and boys desired, but not, in fact, on their sequence.

Table 9.4 presents means and variances for each of the three variables—pregnancies, diagnoses, and corrective abortions—for the set of sequential family goals, as well as the associated probability of needing no corrective abortions. In each case the expected numbers are roughly proportional to total children desired, being simply the sum of the values associated with a single boy or girl. One boy requires 2.35 pregnancies, whereas two boys requires twice as many, 4.71. A girl requires 2.47 pregnancies, so two boys and a girl require 7.18. The same relationship obtains for diagnoses and corrective abortions, and for the variances associated with each. The expected number of corrective abortions approximately equals the number of children desired, whereas diagnoses are roughly twice that number. Because of the small size of post-diagnosis pregnancy loss, θ_2^*, expected corrective abortions is close to expected diagnoses less k. Expected diagnoses equals $1 - (\theta_2 - \theta_2^*) = .85$ times expected pregnancies.

The probability of avoiding any corrective abortions declines sharply as the number of children increases. If a single boy is sought, the probability is

Table 9.4

MEANS AND VARIANCES OF TOTAL PREGNANCIES, DIAGNOSES, AND CORRECTIVE ABORTIONS, BY SEQUENTIAL FAMILY GOAL[a]

Family goal	Mean			Variance			Probability of no corrective abortion
	Pregnancies	Diagnoses	Corrective abortions	Pregnancies	Diagnoses	Corrective abortions	
b	2.35	2.00	.98	3.18	2.00	1.93	.51
g	2.47	2.10	1.07	3.63	2.31	2.23	.48
bb	4.71	4.00	1.95	6.37	4.00	3.86	.26
bg	4.82	4.10	2.05	6.81	4.31	4.16	.24
gg	4.94	4.20	2.15	7.25	4.61	4.46	.23
bbb	7.06	6.00	2.93	9.55	6.00	5.79	.13
bbg	7.18	6.10	3.02	10.00	6.31	6.09	.12
bgg	7.29	6.20	3.13	10.43	6.61	6.39	.12
ggg	7.41	6.30	3.22	10.88	6.92	6.69	.11
bbbb	9.41	8.00	3.90	12.74	8.00	7.72	.07
bbbg	9.53	8.10	4.00	13.18	8.31	8.02	.06
bbgg	9.65	8.20	4.10	13.62	8.61	8.32	.06
bggg	9.76	8.30	4.20	14.06	8.92	8.62	.06
gggg	9.88	8.39	4.30	14.51	9.22	8.92	.05

[a] See Appendix, Section C of Kobrin and Potter (1981) for relevant formulas. Parameter assignments are those cited in Table 9.2.

.51, to be compared with .07 when four boys are desired. As might be expected, a goal favoring boys yields a slightly higher chance of avoiding corrective abortion than an equivalent one which favors girls. Nevertheless, the loads in every case are very high. Any given two-child sequence requires on average more than four diagnoses, about two corrective abortions, and $5-5\frac{1}{2}$ pregnancies. And the variances are extremely high, so that while about one-quarter of the couples would require no abortions, many would require far more than two. A strategy which has some hope of reducing these loads would seem highly desirable. This is what a compositional family goal makes possible.

COMPOSITIONAL GOALS

If some number of children of each sex is desired, and the sequence in which they are born is not important, than a strategy can be followed that greatly reduces the number of diagnoses, abortions, and pregnancies. The abortion-reducing rule depends on the future sex composition wanted in such a way as to allow family formation to proceed without regulation as long as a child of either sex is still wanted. This is true for the first birth trial, based on the overall compositional goal, and continues for each succeeding one until only children of one sex are required to meet the goal. The proportion of birth trials that can go unregulated is greater the greater the number of children of each sex desired and the more balanced the composition preferred.

Table 9.5 displays information on the expected values and variances for pregnancies, diagnoses, and corrective abortions associated with this abortion-reducing strategy. The basic pattern of variation is similar to that achieved as a result of pursuing a sequential goal: Mean corrective abortions are roughly half of mean diagnoses and rise almost in direct proportion to desired family size. Again, for a given family size, they are slightly higher for compositions favoring daughters. The main difference between the two strategies is that the ratios of diagnoses to pregnancies are consistently lower, and often much lower, by virtue of some birth trials being unregulated. To take the most extreme instance considered, for a compositional goal of two girls and two boys the ratio of diagnoses to pregnancies is .46 (3.08 to 6.63) in contrast to .85 (8.20 to 9.65) when all birth trials are being regulated. This large difference arises in the ratio of diagnoses to pregnancies because for a family goal of two of each sex, only 38% of the birth trials need, on average, be regulated under the abortion-reducing rule. The first two trials need never be regulated; only about half the time need the third be regulated (when either two boys or two girls resulted from the first two trials). The last of the four birth trials is always regulated, so the expected proportion regulated is three-eighths, or 38%. Overall, the number of preg-

Table 9.5
MEANS AND VARIANCES OF TOTAL PREGNANCIES, DIAGNOSES, AND CORRECTIVE ABORTIONS AND PROBABILITY OF AVOIDING CORRECTIVE ABORTION BY COMPOSITIONAL FAMILY GOAL[a]

Family goal	Mean			Variance			Probability of no corrective abortion
	Pregnancies	Diagnoses	Corrective abortions	Pregnancies	Diagnoses	Corrective abortions	
bg	3.61	2.05	1.03	3.68	2.17	2.08	.49
bbg	5.35	3.00	1.48	5.56	4.02	3.15	.38
bgg	5.50	3.15	1.60	6.14	4.58	3.62	.36
gbbb	7.39	4.47	2.19	8.44	7.18	4.95	.26
ggbb	6.63	3.08	1.54	6.13	4.29	3.40	.37
gggb	7.68	4.76	2.43	9.73	8.28	5.84	.23

a/ Relevant formulas are found in the Appendix, Section D, of Kobrin and Potter (1981).

nancies is roughly twice the number of desired births. There is about the same number of diagnoses expected as desired births except for the balanced sex, four-child goal, where balance and size combine to limit diagnoses to barely over three. Corrective abortions average about half the number of desired births, except, again, for compositional goals of two boys and two girls, where the abortion load is reduced as well. To illustrate precisely the gain of the abortion-reducing strategy possible for compositional goals relative to the full regulation needed for sequential goals, Table 9.6 shows the ratio of pregnancies, diagnoses, and corrective abortions expected for a compositional goal relative to its respective sequential equivalent. Ratios for the probability of escaping corrective abortion entirely, and the proportions of birth trials regulated, are also shown.

The reduction in diagnostic and abortion loads is clearly substantial. The abortion-reducing strategy requires on average only 38–58% as many diagnoses and corrective abortions. These ratios are governed by the average proportion of birth trials regulated under the abortion-reducing decision rule (last column of Table 9.6). The ratio of pregnancies required is higher, varying between 69 and 79% of those needed for a sequential goal, because during an unregulated birth trial the number of pregnancies is not 0, as it is for diagnoses and corrective abortions, but rather averages $1/(1 - \theta_2)$ or 1.20.

The most dramatic contrast between the two strategies is in the probability of avoiding any corrective abortion. For a two-child family a compositional goal of a boy and a girl will be achievable without recourse to selective

Table 9.6
RATIOS OF EXPECTED NUMBERS OF PREGNANCIES, DIAGNOSES, AND CORRECTIVE ABORTIONS, PROBABILITY OF ESCAPING CORRECTIVE ABORTIONS, AND PROPORTION OF BIRTH TRIALS REGULATED BETWEEN A SEQUENTIAL GOAL AND ITS COMPOSITIONAL EQUIVALENT[a]

Family goal	Pregnancies	Diagnoses	Corrective abortions	Probability of avoiding corrective abortions	Proportion of birth trials regulated
bg	.75	.50	.50	2.03	.50
bbg	.75	.49	.49	3.07	.50
bgg	.75	.51	.51	3.07	.50
gbbb	.78	.55	.55	4.12	.56
ggbb	.69	.38	.38	6.22	.38
gggb	.79	.57	.58	4.12	.57

[a] The first four columns represent ratios of corresponding values of Tables 9.4 and 9.5. Last column values equal $1 - E(z)/k$, k denoting desired family size and the formula for $E(z)$ given in the Appendix Section D of Kobrin and Potter (1981).

abortion more than twice as frequently as a fixed boy–girl (or girl–boy) sequence. The two mixed-sex, three-child goals can be reached more than three times as easily if only composition is required rather than any given sequence of boys and girls. Mixed-sex, unbalanced families of size four (three of one sex, one of the other) are reached more than four times as easily, and a balanced four-child goal (two of each) will avoid selective abortion 6.22 times as frequently as any sequential goal featuring this composition. The amount of abortion reduction, thus, is substantial.

SPACING CONSEQUENCES

The cost of being sure to achieve a sex preference goal, whether of sequence, or only of composition, is clearly high. The cost in terms of diagnoses to achieve a compositional goal averages roughly one for every child desired, and for a sequential goal about two per child. However, amniocentesis as a procedure is perhaps the least problematic of these costs. It is painful, and may be associated with some risk to the fetus, but as discussed this risk is now thought to be extremely low. Abortion costs are quantitatively less, with about one abortion per child expected for sequential goals, and one for every two children for compositional goals. The risks associated with this procedure are higher, but still fairly low. Mortality rates for second trimester abortions are reported to be 15 per 100,000 (Chaudry, Hunt and Wortman 1976).

The number of pregnancies also varies a great deal among unregulated, sequential, and compositional strategies, and this variation imposes costs that should be considered in more detail. As Table 9.6 indicated, although compositional and sequential family goals vary less for pregnancies than for diagnoses or abortions, they still differ appreciably between each other, and differ sharply from a sex indifferent strategy using no regulation at all. Table 9.7 illustrates these contrasts for a popular group of size and sex compositions.

Those who want a two-child family but are indifferent to sex composition and sequence can anticipate 1.20 fewer pregnancies than those who regulate birth trials for a mixed-sex compositional goal, and 2.41 fewer, or half the pregnancies needed for those who regulate each birth trial in order to achieve a mixed-sex sequential goal. For a three-child goal, nearly two to four additional pregnancies can be expected if regulation is used to achieve the most commonly preferred three-child goal of two boys and one girl, and two to five additional pregnancies become necessary to achieve a balanced-sex four-child family.

The results of Table 9.7 assume a spontaneous abortion rate θ_2 of .17. If θ_2 is lowered to .11, supposedly representative of wives in their early twenties, the expected numbers of pregnancies are lowered by a multiplicative factor

Table 9.7
PREGNANCIES EXPECTED BY STRATEGY: SELECTED GOALS[a]

	bg	bbg	bbgg
Unregulated	2.41	3.61	4.82
Regulation for composition	3.61	5.35	6.63
Regulation for sequence	4.82	7.18	9.65

[a] Assumes 1.20 pregnancies per unregulated birth trial. Values for compositional goals and sequential goals are drawn from Tables 9.4 and 9.5.

of roughly $(1.00 - .17)/(1.00 - .11) = .93$. Given a θ_2 – value of .30 that may be considered characteristic of a woman around 40 years of age, the expected number of pregnancies is expanded by a multiplicative factor of approximately $(1.00 - .17)/(1.00 - .30) = 1.19$. Nevertheless, even though the absolute numbers of pregnancies would change, the ratios between pairs of rows in Table 9.7 would be little affected if a θ_2 value of .11 or .30 were substituted for .17.

These additional pregnancies impose a clear cost in terms of time, in addition to the physiological, economic, and emotional costs associated with them. The additional pregnancies are all incomplete, representing corrective abortions as well as some additional spontaneous abortions. Each corrective abortion takes on the average nearly a year, assuming about 6 ovulatory months for conception, 4 months of gestation, and some additional weeks of delay for diagnosing fetal sex and arranging for an abortion. Spontaneous abortions are somewhat less time consuming, but amount to only about one-fifth of the additional pregnancies incurred when the risk of spontaneous abortion is at its average value of .17. This means that the total childbearing period is extended substantially through this method of sex regulation; a couple desiring a three-child family would require on the average 4 years longer to achieve a sequential goal than would one opting for a nonregulated family. Part of this extra time would go into the first-birth trial, so that the age spread between the oldest and youngest child would be less than the total increment, but as a family-building strategy, regulating every birth trial has a substantial impact on expected child spacing.

It would seem that part of this time could be reduced if first-trimester diagnoses were possible. Some research has been directed at finding alternative, less demanding means of sex determination, usually through measurement of fetal hormones (Belisle, Fencl and Tulchinsky 1977). This saves culturing time, but measures taken before the fourteenth gestational week so far are quite unreliable. Even if, however, reliable means of early sex detection were found, the savings would not be great. To begin with, whereas first trimester diagnoses would mean a reduced proportion of early spontaneous abortions, these account for a relatively small fraction of additional pregnancies. Further, for pregnancies with favorable diagnoses, the risk of "late" spontaneous abortion is proportionately increased, which means increased diagnostic and abortion loads. If $\theta_2 = .17$ and if θ_2^*, the incidence of spontaneous abortion that might occur after the first trimester diagnosis is .095 (instead of .020 following midtrimester diagnosis), the quantity $\theta_1 = (1 - \theta_2)/(\theta_2^* + 1 - \theta_2)$ is lowered from .976 to .893. The relevance of θ_1 is that the diagnostic load is to a close approximation proportional to θ_1^{-1} while the corrective abortion load is exactly proportional to θ_1^{-1}.[6] Hence, diagnostic and abortion loads are being increased by a multiplier of $.976/.893 = 1.09$, or about 10%. Thus, the advantage of earlier corrective abortion comes at the price of requiring an enhanced number of them. And as gestation length is a relatively small part of the total time added by an additional corrective abortion, the effects of shorter pregnancies, but more of them, would tend to be offsetting.

The highly variable number of extra pregnancies means that a nontrivial minority of couples could expect to experience extremely long birth-trial sequences, and more yet to experience at least one prolonged birth trial. This not only affects the total time spent in childbearing, but also the birth intervals between children. Usually couples have preferences about birth spacing as well as sex composition. It is plausible, then, that many couples would not tolerate more than a given number of corrective abortions overall or for a given birth interval. After that number of abortions, the couples would be inclined to abandon efforts to preselect the sex of their next child or children and to accept a risk of failing to achieve their original family goal.

SUMMARY

In this chapter, the issue of number control, with its twin problems of subfertility and excess fertility, has been laid aside and attention reserved for the management of sex composition and attendant implications for birth spacing. A basic distinction has been drawn between compositional and sequential goals. The former entails a desired sex composition of children but with indifference about the order in which that composition is realized. A sequential goal by stipulating a single preferred order of sons and daughters sets a more challenging target.

Respecting compositional goals, in the absence of any sex-control technology, there is roughly a 50% chance of realizing a single desired son or a

---

[6] The expected numbers of diagnoses and selective abortions per regulated birth trial are $(h\theta_1)^{-1}$ and $\theta_1^{-1}(1 - h)h^{-1}$, respectively, with $h = .512$ or $.488$ depending on whether a son or a daughter is being sought.

single desired daughter or else a balanced son–daughter composition. The probabilities of realizing a compositional goal by luck alone decreases as the number of children increases, and the decrease is all the more rapid as the objective is made more unbalanced. In the extreme case of an all son or all daughter target, the compositional goal becomes in effect a sequential one with an approximate probability of only $.5^k$ of attaining it, when k is the number of children involved.

None of the current techniques for raising the probability of a boy when a son is wanted or of a girl when a daughter is wanted seem to be efficient enough to elevate appreciably the probabilities of attaining specified compositional goals. This broad approach of trying to augment probabilities of each pregnancy representing the sex wanted at present leaves the odds not greatly changed. In its favor, as its techniques do not require additional pregnancies, it has no adverse consequences for birth spacing.

The very different approach of amniocentesis and selective abortion affords a highly efficient means by which to attain compositional and sequential goals, but at the price of a variably larger number of pregnancies. Besides their direct economic, physical, and emotional costs, these additional interrupted pregnancies impair the couple's control over the spacing of their births. A source of control over sex composition is paid for with a loss of control over birth spacing. To limit this adverse consequence by imposing a low ceiling on the number of diagnoses of fetal sex or of selective abortions is to lower the probability of attaining compositional goals. Nor would development of a reliable first-trimester diagnosis of fetal sex to replace the current midtrimester ones greatly improve the situation. This substitution would not reduce the additional pregnancies, but rather might slightly enhance their number.

It may be concluded, then, that widespread control of sex composition will have to wait on the development of more efficient techniques for raising the probabilities that each pregnancy represents the sex preferred—a state of affairs that does not appear to be in the immediate offing.

REFERENCES

Belisle, S., M. Fencl and D. Tulchinsky (1977), "Amniotic Fluid Testosterone and Follicle-Stimulating Hormone in the Determination of Fetal Sex," *American Journal of Obstetrics and Gynecology, 128* (July), 514–519.

Chaudry, S. L., W. B. Hunt, and J. Wortman (1975), "Pregnancy Termination in Mid-Trimester: Review of Major Methods," *Population Reports,* Series F, No. 5, (Sept.), 65–84.

French, F. E. and J. E. Bierman (1962), "Probabilities of Fetal Mortality," *Public Health Reports, 77* (Oct.), 835–847.

Glass, R. H. (1977), "Sex Preselection," *Obstetrics and Gynecology, 49* (January), 122–126.

Golbus, M. S., W. D. Longham, C. J. Epstein, G. Halbasch, J. D. Stephens, and B. D. Hall (1979), "Prenatal Genetic Diagnosis in 3000 Amniocenteses," *New England Journal of Medicine, 300* (Jan.), 157–163.

Goodman, L. A. (1961), "Some Possible Effects of Birth Control on the Human Sex Ratio," *Annals of Human Genetics, London, 25*, 75–81.

James, W. H. (1975), "Sex Ratio and the Sex Composition of the Existing Sibs," *Annals of Human Genetics, London, 38*, 371–378.

Kobrin, F. E. and R. G. Potter (1981), "Sex Preselection through Amniocentesis and Selective Abortion," in Neil Bennett, Ed., *Sex Selection of Children*, Academic Press (forthcoming).

McDonald, J. (1973), "Sex Predetermination: Demographic Effects," *Mathematical Biosciences, 19*, 137–146.

Malinvaud, E. (1955), "Relations entre la composition des familles et le taux de masculinité," *Journal de la Societé de Statistique de Paris, 96*, 49.

Mason, A. and N. G. Bennett (1977), "Sex Selection with Biased Technologies and Its Effects on the Population Sex Ratio," *Demography, 14* (August), 285–296.

Nortman, D. (1974), "Parental Age as a Factor in Pregnancy Outcome and Child Development," *Reports on Population/Family Planning, 16* (August).

Rinehart, W. (1975), "Sex Preselection not yet Practical," *Population Reports*, Series I, No. 2 (May), 21–32.

Rorvik, D. M. and L. B. Shettles (1970), *Your Baby's Sex: Now you Can Choose*, Dodd Mead, New York.

Sheps, M. C. (1963), "Effects on Family Size and Sex Ratio of Preferences Regarding the Sex of Children," *Population Studies, 17* (July), 66–72.

Smith, D. P. (1974), "Generating Functions for Partial Sex Control Problems," *Demography, 11* (November), 683–689.

Weiler, H. (1959), "Sex Ratio and Birth Control," *American Journal of Sociology*, 298–299.

Williamson, N. E. (1976), *Sons or Daughters: A Cross-Cultural Survey of Parental Preferences*, Sage, Beverly Hills.

Winston, S. (1932), "Birth Control and the Sex Ratio at Birth," *American Journal of Sociology, 38*, 225–231.

Yamamoto, M., T. Ito and G. I. Watanabe (1977), "Determination of Prenatal Sex Ratio in Man," *Human Genetics, 36* (May), 265–269.

Subject Index

B

Bangladesh, 15, 40, 129, 144–148, 152, 153, 164, 165, 176, 178
Basal body temperature (BBT), 32, 36–38, 195, 197
Birth control, see Contraception
Birth defects, see Genetic defects
Birth histories, 23
Birth intervals, 4, 7, 13, 18, 23, 30–31, 87, 117, 237, 143, 148, 152 see also Spacing
  and age, 30–31
  definition of, 44
  duration of, 5, 8, 11, 152
  effect of infant death on, 24
  preferred, 190–195, 199
Birth spacing, see Spacing
Birth trial, 208–209, 220
  probabilities, 211–213
Births, excess, 153, 174–175
Body temperatures, see Basal body temperature
Body weight, 15
Breastfeeding, 7, 8, 10, 16, 17, 21, 23, 24–28, 46, 79, 87, 90, 133, 139, 144, 145
  duration of, 120
  intensity of, 15, 27
  and supplemental feeding, 15, 27
  type of, 27
Bulgaria, 71

C

CBR, see Crude birth rate
Center of Disease Control, 169
Cervical mucus, 197
Chance factors, 127–128, 129, 147–148, 152, 157, 163, 170, 181, 184, 185, 198
Child care, duration of, 182–183
Childbearing, 4, 15
  postponed, 18, 187
  rate of, 5, 12
Childlessness, see Infertility
China, 71
Clomiphene citrate, 197
Coale, A., 22, 82, 101, 138
Cohabitation, 4, 82
Coital frequency, see Intercourse, frequency of
Colombia, 53, 58, 60, 62
Compositional goal, 202, 205, 208, 214, 216–219, 221, 222

Conception, 2
  definition of, 28
  premarital, 28, 175–176, 178
  probability of, 3, 35–38
  rate of, 28–30
  risk of, 3
Conception wait, 5, 7, 28–31, 44, 47, 86, 87, 127, 181
Condom, use of, 70, 187
Contraception, 3, 10, 12, 18, 24, 52, 78
  age-specific, 63–64
  continuity of use, 68
  discontinuation rates, 165–166
  effectiveness of, 5, 18, 65–76, 82–84, 104, 152, 153, 165–169, 170, 174, 176, 177, 178, 186–190
    definitions of, 65, 137, 155
    measures of, 66–76
  failure of, 10, 66–70, 73–76, 166–167, 173–174, 178
  prevalence of, 61–65, 73, 95, 104, 112–113, 117
  reliance on, 154
  trends in, 122–124
  use of, 5, 9, 21, 61–65, 103, 120
Controlled fertility, see Fertility, controlled
Crude birth rate (CBR), 82, 110–112, 118–119
Cuba, 71
Czechoslovakia, 71

D

Diagnostic load, 202, 209, 211, 221
Diaphragm, use of, 70, 74, 187
Diet, see Nutrition
Discontinuation rates, see Contraception, discontinuation rates
Down's syndrome, 207–208

E

Education, 57, 60, 61, 64–65, 73, 112
Europe, 71
Expected value models, 130

F

Family composition, see Sex preselection
Family size, 10, 18, 127, 128, 129, 139, 148, 188–190
  control of, 151–179
Famines, 14, 16–17

STUDIES IN POPULATION

Under the Editorship of: H. H. WINSBOROUGH

Department of Sociology
University of Wisconsin
Madison, Wisconsin

Samuel H. Preston, Nathan Keyfitz, and Robert Schoen. Causes of Death: *Life Tables for National Populations.*

Otis Dudley Duncan, David L. Featherman, and Beverly Duncan. Socioeconomic Background and Achievement.

James A. Sweet. Women in the Labor Force.

Tertius Chandler and Gerald Fox. 3000 Years of Urban Growth.

William H. Sewell and Robert M. Hauser. Education, Occupation, and Earnings: *Achievement in the Early Career.*

Otis Dudley Duncan. Introduction to Structural Equation Models.

William H. Sewell, Robert M. Hauser, and David L. Featherman (Eds.). Schooling and Achievement in American Society.

Henry Shryock, Jacob S. Siegel, and Associates. The Methods and Materials of Demography. *Condensed Edition by Edward Stockwell.*

Samuel H. Preston. Mortality Patterns in National Populations: *With Special Reference to Recorded Causes of Death.*

Robert M. Hauser and David L. Featherman. The Process of Stratification: *Trends and Analyses.*

Ronald R. Rindfuss and James A. Sweet. Postwar Fertility Trends and Differentials in the United States.

David L. Featherman and Robert M. Hauser. Opportunity and Change.

Karl E. Taeuber, Larry L. Bumpass, and James A. Sweet (Eds.). Social Demography.

Thomas J. Espenshade and William J. Serow (Eds.). The Economic Consequences of Slowing Population Growth.

Frank D. Bean and W. Parker Frisbie (Eds.). The Demography of Racial and Ethnic Groups.

Joseph A. McFalls, Jr. Psychopathology and Subfecundity.

Franklin D. Wilson. Residential Consumption, Economic Opportunity, and Race.

Maris A. Vinovskis (Ed.). Studies in American Historical Demography.

Clifford C. Clogg. Measuring Underemployment: Demographic Indicators for the United States.

Doreen S. Goyer. International Population Census Bibliography: *Revision and Update, 1945-1977.*

David L. Brown and John M. Wardwell (Eds.). New Directions in Urban–Rural Migration: *The Population Turnaround in Rural America.*

A. J. Jaffe, Ruth M. Cullen, and Thomas D. Boswell. The Changing Demography of Spanish Americans.

Robert Alan Johnson. Religious Assortative Marriage in the United States.

Hilary J. Page and Ron Lesthaeghe. Child-Spacing in Tropical Africa.

Dennis P. Hogan. Transitions and Social Change: *The Early Lives of American Men.*

F. Thomas Juster and Kenneth C. Land (Eds.). Social Accounting Systems: *Essays on the State of the Art.*

M. Sivamurthy. Growth and Structure of Human Population in the Presence of Migration.

Robert M. Hauser, David Mechanic, Archibald O. Haller, and Taissa O. Hauser (Eds.). Social Structure and Behavior: *Essays in Honor of William Hamilton Sewell.*

Valerie Kincade Oppenheimer. Work and the Family: *A Study in Social Demography.*

Kenneth C. Land and Andrei Rogers (Eds.). *Multidimensional Mathematical Demography.*

John Bongaarts and Robert G. Potter. Fertility, Biology, and Behavior: *An Analysis of the Proximate Determinants.*

In preparation

Randy Hodson. Workers' Earnings and Corporate Economic Structure.

Mary B. Breckenridge. Age, Time, and Fertility: *Applications of Exploratory Data Analysis.*